DASH Diet

Lose Weight Fast and Healthy

By

Aron Smith

Copyright © 2019 Aron Smith

DEDICATION

To all the beautiful, brave souls out there doing their best to live better day after day.

ACKNOWLEDGEMENTS

This book was made possible with the input of some very wonderful people.

I will also like to thank Athena Dumo for her fantastic ability to catch errors where I missed them. You are a proofreader's proofreader. We don't call her "The Eagle" for nothing.

A big thank you to Nick O'Reil Y and Nessa Hol and other wonderful friends of mine who helped out with the other aspects of putting a book out there besides just writing. I'm utterly clueless about these things.

Stan "Titan" Brenner you are a genius and a mad man, and I love you. Thank you for all the amazing ideas!

Gabriel Drinkwater and Esmee Green also deserve honorable mentions. You two pushed me into making this book a reality. In other words, I don't think anyone would be reading this by now if they hadn't put the idea in my head to write about Dash diet. My sincerest thank you to you both!

Table of contents

Introduction

So you're resigned to being a "fatty" for the rest of your life. You've come to accept it. You've come to love your "curves." You've made peace with the extra inches on your frame. You've found coping mechanisms for your thunder thighs forever touching each other with every step you take. You're fine with yourself as you are. Not because you haven't tried. Oh boy, what haven't you tried?

You've purchased every weight loss pill out there. You've gone to the gym religiously. You've tried cardio then weight training. A combo of both, HIIT, LISS, Still nothing.

You've tried every fad diet known to man. You've starved yourself deprived yourself of good nutrition, purchased a lot of sugar-laden "fat-free" products which food companies have continued to push as the better option. Yet where has all this effort taken you? Nowhere. What's all the pain, the suffering, the self-loathing gotten you? Nothing. So, of course, it makes so much sense to just give up and focus on learning to love yourself as you are!

But what if I told you there's a way to the lean body you've only ever dreamed of? What if I told you could finally know what it's like to fit into those size 8 skinny jeans you bought many summers ago to spur you to lose that weight? What if you could finally wear whatever you really want and feel confident no matter what?

Well, there is a way. You ready?

And

It's called the DASH diet.

I know what you're thinking. "Great. Another diet. Way to needlessly lift my hopes up only to "DASH" them against the non-existent rocks of my invisible six-pack abs. I guess this book's just gonna be another door I stop.

I understand. In your shoes, I'd chuck this book into the ocean right after seeing it's about another diet. But hear me out.

The DASH diet is no ordinary diet. It's not just a diet. It's a lifestyle. What do I mean by that? It's a way of eating for life. So you can breathe easy because I'm not going to have you following weird instructions or anything. I'm not going to ask you to eat only boiled eggs and coffee for thirty days. I mean what happens after day 30? Back to business as usual. You go back to eating the way you used to and then the pounds slowly but surely pile back on again.

The DASH way of eating is a lifestyle, which means the end of yoyo dieting for you. All we're going to do is just clean up your usual diet. It's a plan based on simple common sense. We're going to move you away from all the bad stuff - refined sugar cholesterol saturated fat. But it doesn't end there. On the DASH diet, we'll have you focused on eating food that makes your body feel good. You can have fish, low-fat dairy, fruits, vegetables, lean meat, poultry, and whole grains as well. See? No restrictions and a lot of choices!

Above all else, on the DASH diet, you will reduce your sodium intake. This is a great thing if you've got high blood pressure, kidney diseases, diabetes, and osteoporosis. Slashing your salt intake is also something your heart will thank you for - heartily (pun very intended.) You probably want to know why you should bother with this diet. Well, that's what this book will cover. I'm going to help you understand how the DASH diet is crazy easy to follow. More than that, I'm going to show you just how much fat you can burn following this diet and as an added bonus how you can reduce your blood pressure while you're at it.

A caveat though: If you're going to make the DASH diet work, then you need to understand meal planning is key. Once you know what you're going to eat over the coming week, it becomes easier to just automatically eat the right things. You're less likely to cheat since you don't have any room for poor decisions and choices. What this means for you is there will always be lovely delicious meals on hand whenever you're hungry. Plus! You can eat them while watching the fat melt away. I don't know about you, but I think that's a pretty sweet deal.

You might have asked yourself, "Is this diet safe?"

Well, considering that we're going to nix everything that's actually toxic in your diet I'd say a big yes! But don't just take my word for it.

The DASH diet is actually endorsed by the United States Department of Agriculture, the American Heart Association, the US Food and Drug Administration as well as the National Institutes of Health. In fact, across most medical schools, DASH is touted as the best way to eat for you to be at your healthiest. In other words, all of this is based on real actual science and lots of studies.

Feeling better about trying it? Great. Let's get started.

Chapter One What Is The DASH Diet

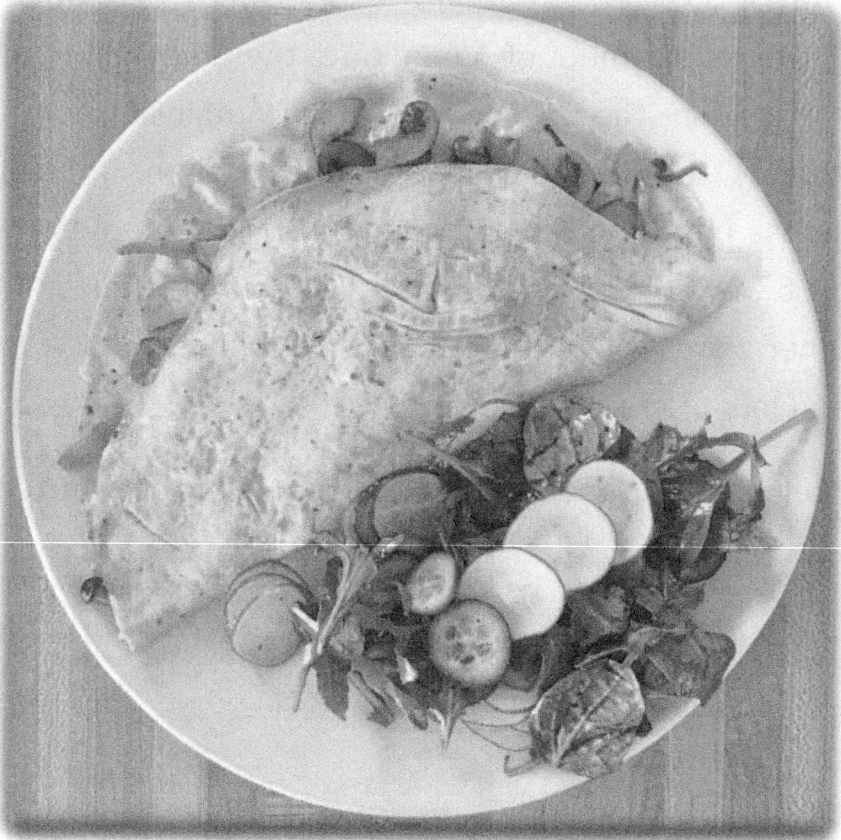

No doubt, you've noticed I've been capitalizing the word "DASH." Yes, it's an acronym. It stands for "Dietary Approaches to Stop Hypertension." You guessed it. This plan wasn't originally set up to be a weight loss diet. Some brilliant researchers from Duke University, School of Medicine, Harvard, Medical School, and Johns Hopkins Medical Center got together to birth this amazing diet. With funding from the National Institutes of Health (NIH), they were able to achieve their goal: to create a diet that would help lower the blood pressure of sufferers of hypertension.

The weight loss effect happened to be some extra delicious icing on the cake. I probably shouldn't be talking about cakes since I'm trying to get you to eat the DASH way.

Besides helping you shed the pounds research has shown that DASH does more than reduce your high blood pressure in just a few weeks. It also results in a significant drop in cholesterol levels, reduces your risk of heart disease and heart failure, some forms of cancer, diabetes, and kidney problems, among other health issues.

Let's Talk About Weight Loss and Maintenance. The truth about weight loss is it's really hard. Add in the fact that we live in times where there's a reduced need to be physically active, and there's glorious sinful food just about everywhere available at the click of your mouse or with just a phone call away, and you can see we've created the perfect environment for obesity to thrive in.

Sure you know you really shouldn't have that extra cookie and sure you know just because it says "Diet insert-name-of-soda-brand-here" doesn't mean it's actually good for you. I'm going to ask you a quick question. If I gave you an option between taking some poison and taking some slightly less poisonous poison wouldn't you look at me as though I'd lost my marbles? Of course!

Because - wonder of wonders - poison is still poison!

However, we live in times where it's okay to indulge.

"Everything in moderation" goes the saying.

"It's called balance," we say tongue-in-cheek. Why does it seem like we're okay with the self-sabotage? With the billions of dollars, Big Food and the quick-fix weight loss industry throw into advertising, it's not hard to see how we're in this dilemma.

Say you actually decide to get off your rhymes-with-pass and do something to lose the weight there's a huge chance your success will be short-lived. Why? Those intense, insane workout programs you happen to see advertised late at night may get you actual results, but they're no good for your body in the long run if you keep up that level of intensity. What about those fad diets? Well, they're not sustainable. Seriously I'll love to see someone try to survive on just boiled eggs and coffee for the rest of their lives. Not only would that be boring and possibly bad for you but goodness gracious what deadly farts you must constantly let out!

So you do the workout programs and follow the diets religiously then lose weight. What happens next? You go back to eating and living like an actual human being in the 2000s and suddenly

"Hello, pot belly, my old friend." In fact, I've seen it happen way more times than I care to count where people get even heavier than they were, to begin with! So what's really going on here?

The reason for this constant nightmare is simple. People don't learn proper eating habits!

This Is Where DASH Saves The Day

With the DASH diet, you can learn eating habits which will serve you for the rest of your life. You can live this way for as long as you breathe and never feel like you're sick and tired of your food options.

This diet is so easy to follow it's ridiculous. All you need to know is just how many calories you need to consume daily and then set up meal plans which will give you those calories. Another great thing is you can find DASH approved food anywhere and everywhere. You don't have to wait several weeks to order your rhubarb unicorn tea from the Upside Down in Hogwarts. Yes, I'm getting my references mixed up. Sue me.

What Makes Up The DASH Diet?

Whole-grain products, Low-fat dairy foods, Fruits, Vegetables, Good fats - the kind you get from nuts. Where red meats and animal fats make an appearance, you need to keep them as low as possible. As for sugar? Should it be in the diet? I'll give you a couple of seconds to figure out the answer. (Hint: No.)

If this sounds like something, you already know because your mom told you over and over again that this was the right way to eat, I wouldn't blame you. DASH is a different animal, though.

Studies have shown the precise combo of servings you need from each food group per day.

These servings largely will be determined by your size and the number of calories you need.

Another thing to factor in is that with the DASH diet, you absolutely must cut your salt intake.

This is non-negotiable. You may want to argue with this but keep in mind that out of all the ridiculous sometimes even dangerous fad diets out there this is the one diet which is backed by the scientific community. If there's one thing I know about scientists, they're never wrong. Well mostly. You can rest assured they aren't wrong about the efficacy of the DASH diet though. A little Googling and you'll see some research which was conducted with 18000 test subjects in a program called "DASH for Health" proved that this diet is the diet to end all others.

The DASH diet is tailor-made to suit you. Are you constantly sitting at a desk from 9 to 5? Then there's a DASH meal plan for you. Do you spend a lot of your time exerting yourself physically?

There's a plan for you too. What about the food? DASH places supreme importance on eating foods with high volume, which are low in calories. In other words, the food may look like a lot but will have a lot fewer calories than you'd expect. It's the difference between eating 100 grams of lettuce (15 calories) and 100 grams of chocolate (546 calories). The best part? You'll be fuller after having the former than the latter. What does this mean? Weight loss over time.

Another focus of the DASH diet is eating foods which make you "work." I don't know about you, but eating can be a lot of work. All that chewing! Gah! Hear me out, though. With the DASH diet, you'll have foods which take a lot more time for you to chew Why is that? The tougher the food is, the more time you'll need to chew it. The more time you take to chew it, the more likely you'll get that "full feeling" before you're even done!

So let's summarize this bad boy, shall we?

You need food which will practically fill your stomach, so you feel completely satisfied.

You need the food to be low in calories despite how much it is in volume.

You need the food to take you a fair amount of time to eat. This way your gut is likely to signal your brain that it's full before you're even done!

What about foods with high density? You know all that good sweet red meat and that rich, full -fat cheese and don't even let us get started on Almighty Chocolate? Ooh and delicious pastries?

I'm going to sound like a broken record here but if you want results, keep them to an absolute minimum. Yes, you can have some of this on the diet but for best results just lay off of them. It's really up to you. Nothing's completely out of bounds. Except for Sugar. You can go sit in the corner and think about all the things you've done wrong.

Why You Should Start DASH-ing.

With DASH you'll lose weight, and in the long term, you'll successfully keep it. Since there's going to be a lot of fiber in your DASH meal plan, you'll find that your food stays in your gut much longer, so you stay feeling full for a while and only with a few calories! What this means is that you'll inevitably find yourself eating fewer calories than you need daily. Hello, weight loss! In fact, you'll be so full you most likely won't be able to eat as much or as often as the DASH diet requires you to (5 - 6 times a day).

Another good thing DASH has got going for it is your energy levels stay up for much longer than if you were on a SAD diet, for instance. You won't find yourself desperate for some junk food which spikes your insulin willy nilly and then plunges it leaving you ridiculously tired. You know that slump you experience after your lunch break? Well with DASH you can say goodbye to that. You'll have so much boundless energy you could take over from the Energizer bunny.

DASH is super easy to follow. You can have all the good food you love. You know what happens when you're on other silly fad diets? You begin to feel deprived. That causes you to desperately seek out all the bad food you shouldn't just so you can stuff your face. When you give in to that feeling caused by the deprivation, you feel even worse. You don't have to worry about this with DASH since you have a whole lot of variety to work with.

Following the DASH diet doesn't leave you at risk. Like I've already mentioned every medical institution of high repute already recommends this particular diet. You're definitely not risking your health when you follow this wholesome way of eating. In fact, it's been found that this style of eating has a more potent effect on the reduction of blood pressure and in improving heart health than any pill out there. You don't always need to take meds. They have a ton of side effects which can be detrimental. Thank goodness for the dudes who came up with DASH right?

Now some doctors recommend this diet instead of pills. One more reason to DASH.

Finally, DASH is free. You don't need to buy that workout program with the fancy meal boxes.

You don't need to shell out thousands of dollars for

another protein shake or for some magic pill that will melt all your fat away. Don't buy into that stuff. They don't work Unless they were made by unicorns. Since we are yet to actually spot a real-life unicorn - I shouldn't have to repeat myself

- They just don't work. With DASH, you can eat healthily, lose weight, improve your cholesterol levels, and more all for free.

Scientific Studies on the DASH Diet It only makes sense that I refer you to studies which show how effective the DASH diet is in helping you lose weight and get healthy. So let's get into it.

As I've already mentioned before the DASH diet was created in order to reduce the blood pressure in hypertension sufferers. Hypertension happens to be so severe that in the Seventh Report of the Joint National Committee on Prevention Detection Evaluation and Treatment of High Blood Pressure (2002) hypertension was said to affect at least 1 billion people worldwide.

This alone was a good reason to look for a solution. Why? High blood pressure puts you at risk of other cardiovascular diseases such as heart attacks, strokes, and even kidney diseases. This is according to the National Heart, Lung, and Blood Institute (NHLBI).

Using a randomized control trial (RTI), the NHLBI, along with five top-notch medical research centers in the United States, conducted a DASH study in 1992. Till this point, it's still one of the largest studies ever conducted and one of the most detailed ones as well.

To make the foods more accessible to every John and Jane out there (if it proved successful), the study made a meal plan that was made up of everyday foods. Between August 1993 and July 1997, this premier DASH study was carried out. Since there was already research which showed an increase in certain dietary minerals and fiber leads to reduced blood pressure. It was with this premise that the study was carried out.

During the study, there were three diets. One, the control which followed the usual American diet and was severely missing important minerals like potassium, magnesium, and calcium as well as low in fiber. Another diet was similar to the control but simply had a lot more fruits and veggies with fewer snacks and sweet treats. The final diet was the DASH diet, which had an increase of fruits and veggies as well as low-fat dairy. It also had a reduction in fat, especially saturated fat. The protein and fiber levels were also significantly higher than in the control diet.

At the end of the study, it was found that there was a significant decrease in blood pressure in subjects who followed the DASH diet compared to subjects who followed the first two diets we mentioned. The study showed this reduction in blood pressure within 2 weeks from when the DASH subjects began their diet.

By the end of this study, there was a follow-up study called the "DASH-Sodium study." The purpose was to see if the DASH diet could yield even more benefits when adhered to with low sodium intake. The researchers were also curious as to what effects varying levels of sodium intake might have on the subjects. This study lasted from September 1997 to November 1999 and involved 412 test subjects all with prehypertension or stage 1 hypertension. These two groups were randomly assigned to various groupings. Along with the control diet (typical American diet), there was the DASH diet with three further distinctions by sodium level: 1500 mg/day, 2400 mg/day or 3000 mg/day of sodium.

The end of this study showed there was a reduction in blood pressure once the subjects assigned to DASH began their diet. It also showed that the effect of sodium in subjects on the control diet was even more potent than in subjects on the DASH diet. In the three versions of the DASH diet, it was revealed that the group with the least amount of sodium obtained the best results in reducing blood pressure.

Another study carried out in 2010 which is worthy of note is the Effects of the DASH Diet Alone and in Combination With Exercise and Weight Loss on Blood Pressure and Cardiovascular Markers in Men and Women with High Blood Pressure by James A. Blumenthal Ph.D., Michael A. Babyak Ph.D., and Alan Hinderliter MD et al.

This study set out to see what happens when you just

follow the DASH diet versus what happens when you incorporate exercise. Participants were also prehypertensive or with stage 1 hypertension. They were also obese or at least overweight.

The study concluded that while there was weight loss all round as well as a reduction in blood pressure, the subjects with the most notable decrease in blood pressure were those who incorporated some exercise.

There are many more studies out there, which show time after time that the DASH diet is the best diet there is. In fact, just in 2018 the U.S. News and World Report placed the Dash diet as the number one diet out of a list of 40 other reviewed diets - for the eighth time. Even better? It's been at the top of the list for 8 years consecutively.

So what can we glean from this? Following the DASH-style of eating with a reduced intake of sodium and increased physical activity is a surefire way to not just lose weight fast but to get healthy as well.

Chapter Two Putting DASH to Work

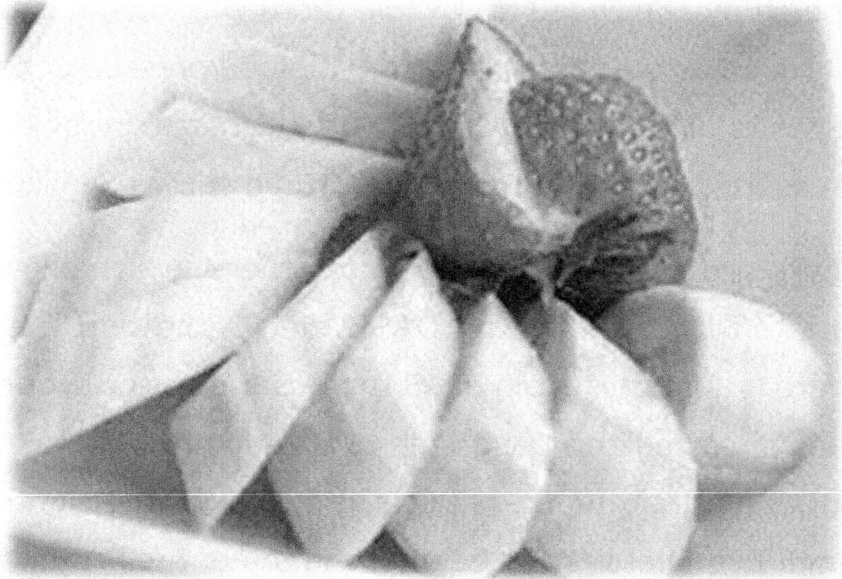

The great thing about the DASH diet is you're going to find it way easier than anything else you've tried. We're going to channel all our energy towards foods we want to have. The last thing I want you to do is drain yourself by focusing on what you should avoid eating. Get it?

Now the way we're going to handle this, you won't have to count calories. I personally hate counting calories. It's one of the things that just makes weight loss a burden. I can't imagine how people need to measure their food ever so precisely and methodically before eating it. It's not hard to see how you could give up before you've even hit a week of doing this!

What are we going to do instead? We're going to pay attention to how balanced our food is.

That's it. We want to be sure each food group is represented in balance.

That out of the way we're going to split your DASH action plan into two distinct stages. Now I'm not going to lie Stage One is going to be a heck of a lot more restricted than Stage Two, but in the end, this is how you're going to achieve incredible results following DASH. I don't know about you, but results are very addictive. Once you start to see your favorite pair of jeans or yoga pants get way too loose for comfort, you'll find you're even more motivated to keep up the good work!

DASH Diet Habits

You're going to learn to have a lot of veggies. Yes, you're going to eat your greens. Don't worry, there are lots of ways to make them delicious! I personally think they already are just super.

Vegetables will make up most of what's on your plate.

Another habit you're going to pick up is eating a lot of foods that are rich in protein. Why? They help you stay sated for longer. What this implies is you're less likely to want to snack in-between your meals. Also, your blood sugar will be at the most optimum level since you're not eating so much starch and sugar anymore. Another great thing about this is your metabolism gets a lovely boost! Rather than have your insulin erratically spiking and dropping all over the place because of sugars and starch, you'll require a lot less insulin when you eat the DASH way.

Do you suffer from Irritable Bowel Syndrome or other digestive issues? Within just a few days you'll notice you have fewer symptoms! To top it all off, you'll see your belly shrink in only a matter of days. No, I'm not exaggerating. I mean days. Once the positive eating habits you get from DASH take hold you're going to not just reach your weight loss goal but also maintain your new healthy weight effortlessly.

Now a caveat: if you're on medication for diabetes and blood pressure you need to speak with your doctor before you jump on this diet okay? Because you're going to find that following this plan will make you need less of your medication. I want to make it extremely clear that you must not change anything about your medication without first seeing your doctor even if the benefits of following the DASH diet makes it seem like it's time to come off the meds.

For some people who are dealing with weight problems, it's not all necessarily down to a sedentary lifestyle and an incredibly horrible diet. Sometimes it's an issue with dysmetabolic syndrome also known as

Syndrome X. In women with weight loss issues, they could be sufferers of polycystic ovarian syndrome which you probably know of as PCOS. Sufferers of PCOS are also affected by Syndrome X dealing with a bunch of stuff like high levels of fat and sugar in the blood high blood pressure really thick waistlines and even low HDL levels.

If this is you right now, I can only imagine what it must be like for you going through all this. The good news, though, is that the DASH diet actually helps you fix all these problems!

DASH Approved Foods for Stage One

Here are the foods you can have on the DASH diet in moderate servings: High-Protein Low Saturated Fat Foods

Lentils soybeans

Non-fat and/or low-fat cheese

Lean meat poultry fish

Eggs and/or egg substitutes

Yogurt (unsweetened is better, but you can have some artificially sweetened yogurt once a day) Protein-Packed Foods and Healthy Fats

Fatty fish

Seeds and nuts (unsalted nuts are best. Also unroasted nuts are preferable) Heart-Friendly Fats

Vegetable oils (canola and olive oils in particular) Nut oils (no palm oil and no coconut oil. These two have high saturated fat levels) Vegetable and nut oil-based salad dressings

You can have as much of non-starchy vegetables as you like - except for corn potatoes and such. You may also have as much sugar-free gelatin as you like! Go on and enjoy them as great substitutes for your deserts and fruits.

Foods to Avoid

Alcohol (Obviously)

Caffeinated drinks (You may have some along with a snack or a meal) Milk

All sugary foods (Yes that includes fruit)

Starchy foods (You may have beans, but you most certainly cannot have bread rice potatoes pasta batter-fried foods and such).

How to Kick Ass on The DASH Diet

I'm going to give you a roadmap to success on this diet, okay? If you follow this religiously, I promise soon you'll have to go shopping for some new clothes. Smaller clothes.

Get to bed early.

When you begin Stage One, you'll find your energy levels a bit out of whack. You'll get tired a lot earlier than you're used to. Don't panic. It's completely natural. I promise in a couple of weeks your energy levels will be reset, and you'll feel good as new Don't skip meals.

Don't skip your snacks either. Yes, I know it would seem like if you skipped a meal here and there it would really kick the fat loss into gear. Don't do it, though. If you do your blood sugar levels will plummet, and you'll find yourself hungrier than a bear after a thousand-year winter. You'll also feel super shaky and possibly light-headed. No good. Plus you want to master your hunger and the only way to do that is learning to keep your blood sugar on a level.

Get your fluids.

Remember those proverbial eight glasses of water a day? You're going to need them. Stage One of the DASH diet - which lasts 2 weeks - will dehydrate you if you don't get that water in. Add to that the fact that since you're not taking in as much starch and crap sugar in your system, your body no longer has any reason to hold on to excess fluid. So get that water in.

Get a bit of salt in.

Yes, you read, right. Let me explain. In this first stage, you need just a bit of salt. Why? To stop your body from flushing out all the fluid. Dehydration is dangerous, but so is overhydration. Also when you're drinking eight glasses a day, you're going to lose a fair bit of electrolytes which doesn't feel good believe me.

The salt will keep you from feeling like utter crap.

Keep exercise under or at 30 minutes. No more than that not during Stage One. Keep it light-to-moderate. If you decide you'll like to channel your inner beast in a workout, you'll find your blood sugar levels will drop way-way down. You don't even need to work out during Stage One. However, walking is excellent for burning belly fat. So take walks. The best thing? You won't lose muscle walking.

Relax. It's not uncommon to feel out of sorts when you're in Stage One. You might get super irritable. You might find yourself getting angry at the silliest things like "Why the heck is this floor on the floor?!" Just breathe through it. Your body is simply trying to adapt to the changes you're making. When you feel yourself getting overly emotional pause, close your eyes, take deep relaxing breaths, and gently remind yourself, "This too shall pass." It is only a phase. No more.

So breathe through it and relax.

Take pictures.

Before you start strip down to your birthday suit or at least your skivvies and take pictures. Don't take them looking for evidence that what you're doing is working. Just take them. I promise before Stage One is up, you'll see reasons to keep going. Keeping track of your progress is a great way to stay on track. I'm not a fan of the scales seeing as a lot could make them fluctuate. But pictures never lie. The way your body fits in your clothes (and out of them!) will tell the story over time.

Keep the end in sight.

There will be times you wonder why the heck you started this in the first place. There will be times that Hershey's bar looks so so good. There will be times when the smell of your cousin's pizza taunts you. You feel like if you could take one bite, your soul would be healed. In times like this, remember why you started.

Stage One Food Suggestions

I'm going to get into a lot more detail about what to eat for each day of Stage One, but before I do, I figured I'll give you a rough idea of what kind of meals you'll be having over the next 2 weeks.

What's for Breakfast?

1 or 2 slices of ham or bacon. You can also choose soy options if available.

Eggs or egg substitutes which you may have with some cheese.

V8 juice or just tomato juice.

Unsweetened yogurt. Artificially sweetened yogurt is fine too.

Pre-lunch Snacks

You can have at least 2 of the following snacks: Low-fat cheese. You can opt for some light string cheese or some light cottage cheese. The kind that's 4 ounces.

¼ cup of nuts or even less. If you want some cheese with your nuts, then you can only have one tablespoon of nuts.

Vegetables. Celery, cucumbers, peppers (sliced), radishes, carrots cherry, and tomatoes will work great.

Lunch Time!

Here you get to pick a high-protein meal and slap on all the other side dishes.

Roll-ups. You can use lettuce turkey ham or lean roast beef as a wrap with some low-fat cheese.

A salad with a wide array of vegetables and some protein as well. No breadcrumbs and definitely no croutons. Use light cheese. Once in a while, you may use regular cheese.

Tomatoes with salad. The salad could be chicken or tuna or egg or egg whites or a mix of some or all of them.

Jell-O. Definitely the sugar-free kind.

Post-lunch Snacks

You can have these after lunch and shortly before dinner as well. They're the same as the pre-lunch snacks, but you can add on:

Jell-O (Sugar-free artificial y sweetened)

Salad with vegetable-oil based dressing.

Non-starchy vegetables.

Strips of pepper dipped in hummus guacamole or a vegetable-oil based salad dressing.

Peanuts. (Still in the shell. Don't go above 20 peanuts.) Of course, this plan presupposes you have complete control over everything you eat but what happens when you need to eat out for lunch because of work or hang out with friends for dinner?

Eating Out

Breakfasts

Omelets or eggs

Bacon. Don't go overboard.

Tomato juice. Keep it low-sodium. Have no more than 6 ounces.

Sliced tomatoes. They're the perfect substitute for toast and potatoes.

Lunch

Salads with lean high-protein food.

Bunless burgers or chicken combined with a salad or some coleslaw on the side. No fries.

Dinner

Fish, poultry, or lean meat.

Salad with vegetable oil-based dressing.

Some veggies.

No sugary dessert. Sorry kids. But! There's always that sugar-free Jell-O!

When Grocery Shopping for Stage One...

These are things you should definitely make sure you stock up on Eggs and/or egg substitutes. They may or may not have veggies in them.

Sugar-free Jell-O

Guacamole

Hummus

Tuna, salmon, and other fatty fish. You can get the canned ones for convenience.

Light cheeses (string cheese, cottage cheese, individually packed).

Ground sirloin. Make sure it's extra lean.

Turkey breasts

De-skinned chicken breasts

Seafood. Nothing fried.

Nuts. Get the kind still in its shell since dealing with shells means you won't eat as much as you would if you could just pop them in your mouth straight away. Also, make sure your nuts aren't oil-roasted. Dry roast is better. You can also get raw cashews, almonds, and walnuts.

Fresh vegetables: summer squash, zucchini, baby carrots, fresh peppers, lettuce, radishes, tomatoes, and so on.

Frozen vegetables: cauliflower, green beans, green peas, spinach, broccoli, Brussels sprouts mixed veggies, and so on.

Remember this: you only need to pick the foods you like. Don't force yourself to eat stuff you absolutely hate just because it's on the list.

It is really important that you have a plan of action if you're going to succeed. I mean sure you can buy all the food you need but how do you make sure you only ever eat that instead of some delicious Dunkin Donuts? You need a plan.

First of all, you want to always have access to DASH-approved foods. Keep them handy that way if you start to feel peckish because a co-worker decided today was the perfect day to bring back a slice of pizza from lunch you can reach for your DASH food instead.

Speaking of work, make sure you pack your lunches and your snacks. Take them to work. Keep your office fridge stocked with your food or find a way to store them in a bag.

Make sure you plan your meals in advance. Snacks too. Once you have a plan, it's easier to execute.

You can't skip your meals or snacks. I know I've already mentioned this before, but it's really vital, so you don't slide down that slippery slope caused by low blood sugar.

You can do some meal prep ahead of time, so it's easier for you to cook your meals quickly. For instance, you can boil and peel a lot of eggs put them in a Ziploc bag and store in your refrigerator. You could make some chili, so you have it handy to make other meals. Try grilling some chicken breasts, so you have them handy for your salad or other meals.

Dining out? Before you leave, be sure to check what the restaurant offers and plan accordingly before you go. Trust me it's better to do this before you get to the restaurant than to wait until you're there and staring at some guy's delicious plate of pasta.

Above all else, keep the end in sight, and you will succeed.

DASH Diet Stage One Daily Servings

You may have a different idea of food combinations to opt for when on the DASH diet. So rather than giving you heavy-handed rules I'm going to create a simple little guide to help you figure out the basics of what you should eat and how much of it.

FATS

Small appetite:

1 - 2 ounces.

Medium appetite:

2 - 3 ounces.

Big appetite:

2 - 4 ounces.

DAIRY

Small appetite:

2 ounces.

Medium appetite:

2 - 3 ounces.

Big appetite:

2 - 4 ounces.

SEEDS NUTS BEANS

Small appetite:

1 ounce.

Medium appetite:

1 - 2 ounces.

Big appetite:

1 - 2 ounces.

EGGS, POULTRY, FISH, AND LEAN MEAT

Small appetite:

5 - 6 ounces.

Medium appetite:

6 - 8 ounces.

Big appetite:

8 - 11 ounces.

VEGETABLES (NON-STARCHY)

Small appetite:

5 - unlimited ounces

Medium appetite:

5 - unlimited ounces.

Big appetite:

5 - unlimited ounces.

DASH STAGE ONE GOALS

During or by the end of Stage One, you'll have realized how easy it is to get a load on your hunger when your blood sugar isn't all over the place.

You'll have successfully soothed the way your body responds to your past overindulgence in food, particularly excess calories from starch and sugar.

You'll have made a habit of preparing your meals colorful with all sorts of veggies as well as partnering them with fish, poultry, lean meats, and other high protein foods, including low-fat dairy.

Your body will quit producing way too many triglycerides LDL cholesterol and insulin, which triggers it to store fat. So you're going to melt the pounds away and feel like a bazillion buck!

You'll have successfully implemented a healthy way of eating, which will prolong and increase the quality of your life. Score!

ACTION PLAN FOR THE DASH DIET

Grab a post-it note, and in writing promise yourself, you'll commit to the DASH diet. Stick it up on the fridge where you'll see it every day.

Commit to going grocery shopping for DASH foods only.

Identify what new DASH foods you'll be adding to your diet.

Identify which of the DASH foods are absolute favorites for you so you can reward yourself with them when you pull through each day or week.

Identify the challenges you might have to face, which could ruin your chances of sticking with the diet.

Make a plan of action for how you'll deal with said challenges and commit to following through.

Chapter Three DASH Diet Stage One: Meal Plans

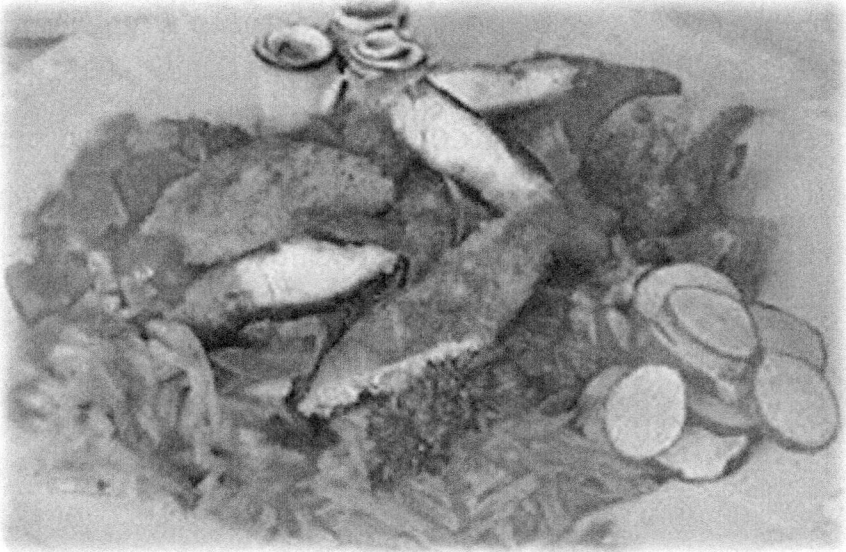

Alright, it's time to kick your body's metabolism into high gear! I've already given you everything you need to know about Stage One of the DASH diet in the previous chapter. Now we're going to take a look at a Stage One meal plan I've put together for you to follow. Again nothing is set in stone; you can mix and match as you need to. I'm fairly certain you're going to find new interesting ways to create your DASH meals!

Feel free to substitute foods which are similar to one another. You can also go ahead and repeat certain days if they're easier for you to follow or you just find those meals tastier. Don't like a certain day's plan? Scrap it all together and opt for a different plan - as long as it's still DASH of course.

Keep in mind that you want to have as much of the filling foods as you can along with the high protein foods. Anytime you feel a tad light-headed grab another snack if you already had one before.

Let's Talk Portions

When your plate is piled high and wide with vegetables, you're going to find yourself incredibly sated after every meal. You could never have way too much non-starchy veggies. Unless your stomach happens to have the capacity of a silo in which case my bad.

AS for poultry, fish, and lean meats, make sure the portion is no bigger than your hand. Obviously, if you're a big guy or girl, you're going to have big hands. This is fine. Just don't go beyond that size. Generally, men need more protein than the fairer sex but on the DASH diet, whatever your gender or size just keep it to the size of a hand and no more.

Let's Talk Appetite

During Dash Stage One, you'll find your appetite decreases over time. So it's okay to stop eating when you feel you've had enough.

If shortly after eating you start to feel quite hungry, then there's a huge chance it's because your serving size is way too small. Particularly the protein. So you can fix that by slightly upping the protein.

Bear in mind that you're going to be a bit bored toward

the end of Stage One. It's not unusual.

Actually, it's a good thing if you find yourself bored because chances are you won't go overboard with your eating since your appetite is so... Meh.

But Where's The Fruit?

Yes, I love fruit too. I understand how you feel. But that's what the sugar-free Jell-O is for. You get to have that with most of your lunches and dinners since they're quite refreshing, super low in calories, and very satisfying.

We can't have fruit right now because fruit is going to spike your insulin Also with Jell-O you can have about two to three with each lunch and/or dinner without worrying about taking in too many calories! Jell-O comes in so many flavors so be sure to try as many as you can to avoid boredom. You'll come to love Jell-O. I promise. And when you do have fun!

Speaking of flavors, light yogurt has an amazing variety too. So don't limit yourself. Make this an adventure in taste.

Making This Easy for You

I know not everyone loves to cook. With that in mind, I've given you a number of foods which will only take a small amount of prep time. Pre-packaged veggie mixes are more than ideal for making your salads, for instance. You have so much variety. You could choose bagged mixes like a spring mix a coleslaw blend a romaine mix or an iceberg mix. You could opt for broccoli slaw or grated carrots. You could mix and match the combinations. It's like building stuff with Legos.

Have fun with this!

Conversely, you could just hit up a salad bar and get your salad in no time along with some boiled eggs.

You're going to find a lot of eggs and egg substitutes in this plan I've drawn up. It's important that you choose really good eggs which pack a lot of omega-3 fatty acids. This kind is really low in cholesterol. Don't worry about having so many eggs. They're good for you.

Let's Talk Drinks

Here are your choices: diet sodas tea (artificially sweetened or unsweetened) black coffee and of course the all -important water. No, you may not have alcohol since some alcoholic drinks have sugar, and all alcoholic beverages definitely have a lot of calories. Also, alcohol is not your friend. It's a disinhibitor. In other words, if you have a drink, you're likely to find ways to convince yourself that a burger with fries and a large coke is actually a DASH food on a metaphysical level or something.

Alright, let's hop to it!

Meal Plan for DASH Diet Stage One

Day 1

Breakfast

An omelet and 4 - 6 ounces of low sodium tomato juice.

Pre-Lunch Snack

Some baby carrots and 1 stick of light cheese

Lunch

Fried chicken breast (no skin no breading); coleslaw some baby carrots; and some sugar-free Jell-O

Post-Lunch Snack

4 ounces of fat-free artificially sweetened yogurt; and 18 cashews Pre-Dinner Snack (can be skipped)

Guacamole (2 ounces); and some crunchy pepper strips.

Dinner

Grilled chicken; salad with Italian dressing or vegetable oil-based dressing; add in some mixed veggies (microwaved or steamed); and sugar-free Jell-O

Day 2

Breakfast

A hard-boiled egg, 1 bacon (2 tops) with some tomato juice (6 ounces tops and please make it low-sodium)

Pre-Lunch Snack

Grape tomatoes (6); and 1 wedge of light cheese Lunch

Turkey-Swiss roll-ups with cheese and/or lettuce as the wrap and deli turkey slices as meat.

(2-3); some coleslaw (½ - 1 cup); snow peas (raw) or sugar snap pea pods (have as much as you prefer); sugar-free Jell-O

Post-Lunch Snack

Baby carrots and 1 stick of light cheese

Pre-Dinner Snack (can be skipped)

20 single peanuts still in the shell

Dinner

Carrots and onions sautéed in vegetable oil; salad with vegetable oil-based dressing or Italian dressing; Jell-O

Day 3

Breakfast

Bacon (1 - 2 slices); with eggs (scrambled); and some cranberry juice (4 - 6 ounces) Pre-Lunch Snack

23 almonds; and light nonfat artificially sweetened yogurt (4 ounces)

Lunch

Tuna salad; side salad with Italian dressing and/or vegetable oil-based dressing Some cherry tomatoes;

and one cup of Jell-O (sugar-free artificially sweetened) Post-Lunch Snack

Light cheese (1 to 2 wedges); and grape tomatoes (6) Pre-Dinner Snack (can be skipped)

Pepper strips dipped in guacamole

Dinner

Sliders (make them bunless and ramp up the flavor with your preferred spices); side salad dressed in balsamic vinegar; broccoli (1 cup); and sugar-free Jell-O (1 - 2)

Day 4

Breakfast

Turkey-Swiss roll-up (turkey from 1 - 2 ounces) with 2% Swiss cheese as wrap Low-sodium tomato juice (4 - 6 ounces)

Pre-Lunch Snack

Chunky peanut butter (2 tablespoons); and 8 baby

carrots Lunch

20 walnuts; grilled chicken and salad; and a sugar-free Jell-O

Post-Lunch Snack

Celery sticks and 1 light string cheese stick

Pre-Dinner Snack (can be skipped)

Pepper strips dipped in hummus

Dinner

1 cup of peas (can be frozen peas heated up in the microwave); ¼ rotisserie chicken; side salad with Italian or vegetable oil-based dressing; and sugar-free Jell-O

Day 5

Breakfast

An omelet; and 4 to 6 ounces diet cranberry juice.

Pre-Lunch Snack

Baby carrots and 1 wedge of light cheese

Lunch

Provolone cheese and roast beef roll-ups with cheese and/or lettuce for the wrap and mustard (or mayo) as a condiment if required; Italian coleslaw (get the already-bagged kind or simply grate some carrots and add thin strips of red pepper) dressed with Italian or vegetable oil and vinegar-based dressing; sliced tomatoes; and a Jell-O cup (sugar-free) Post Lunch Snack

Strawberry-banana light yogurt (artificially sweetened and non-fat) with 10 cashews Pre-Dinner Snack (can be skipped)

20 pistachios (still in shell to slow you down) Dinner

Sautéed skinless chicken breasts with tomato sauce;

a Caprese salad; and a sugar-free Jell-O cup

Day 6

Breakfast

Hard-boiled eggs (1 - 2); bacon (1 slice); and tomato juice (4 - 6 ounces low in sodium) Pre-Lunch Snack

1 wedge of light cheese and grape tomatoes

Lunch

Sliced tomatoes; salmon salad; side salad with Italian or vegetable oil-based dressing; and a sugar-free Jell-O cup

Post-Lunch Snack

Non-fat artificially sweetened key limelight yogurt, and baby carrots Pre-Dinner Snack (can be skipped)

10 peanuts still in shell

Dinner

Spinach; mashed potatoes spiced to your taste with dressing of your choice; grilled chicken; a large tossed salad (tossed with vegetable oil and vinegar or Italian or balsamic dressing) and a sugar-free Jell-O cup

Day 7

Breakfast

Hard-boiled eggs; cashews (10); and tomato juice (4 - 6 ounces low in sodium)

Pre-Lunch Snack

1 light string cheese stick and some baby carrots Lunch

Buffalo chicken salad (you may have this at a restaurant. Go with the grilled option, not the fried) and a sugar-free Jell-O cup

Post-Lunch Snack

Pineapple upside down cake like yogurt (non-fat artificially sweetened) and 10 almonds Pre-Dinner

Snack (can be skipped)

Celery sticks with guacamole

Dinner

Vegetable chili with some shredded cheese (light) and onions if you wish; as well as our favorite sugar-free Jell-O cup

Day 8

Breakfast

Reduced-fat cottage cheese (4 ounces) and diet cranberry juice Pre-Lunch Snack

Strawberry shortcake light yogurt (non-fat artificially sweetened)

Lunch

A cheeseburger without the bun; some broccoli; side salad with Italian dressing or vegetable oil-based dressing; a sugar-free Jell-O cup

Post-Lunch Snack

1 light string cheese stick and 20 walnuts

Pre-Dinner Snack (can be skipped)

Raw veggies (cut) with some light ranch dip

Dinner

Pan-seared salmon with Cajun seasoning mix (the salt-free kind); onions and pepper sautéed in olive oil; side salad with Italian dressing or oil and vinegar-based dressing; a sugar-free Jell-O cup

Day 9

Breakfast

A small cheese omelet with diet cranberry juice (4 - 6

ounces) Pre-Lunch Snack

Light string cheese sticks (1 - 2) with baby carrots (8) Lunch

2 - 3 turkey and Swiss roll-ups with cherry tomatoes coleslaw and sugar-free Jell-O

Post-Lunch Snack

Nonfat artificial y sweetened light yogurt with 10 cashews Pre-Dinner Snack (can be skipped)

Pepper strips with ¼ cup of guacamole or hummus **Dinner**

Green beans spicy pork chops along with some Brussels sprouts (can be roasted) with dressing of your choice; a side salad with oil and vinegar or Italian dressing and sugar-free artificially sweetened Jell-O

Day 10

Breakfast

Boiled eggs (1 - 2) with some Canadian bacon and

low-sodium tomato juice (4 - 6 ounces) Pre-Lunch Snack

1 wedge of light cheese with grape tomatoes

Lunch

Pepper strips chicken salad topped with sesame seeds and sugar-free Jell-O

Post-Lunch Snack

Non-fat or reduced-fat cottage cheese (4 ounces) with celery sticks Pre-Dinner Snack (can be skipped)

Hummus with raw veggies

Dinner

A hearty-sized salad with a wide variety of veggies; some no-crust pizza; and sugar-free artificially sweetened Jell-O

Day 11

Breakfast

An omelet with diet cranberry juice (4 - 6 ounces) Pre-Lunch Snack

Peanut butter with celery or carrot sticks

Lunch

Roast beef and Swiss cheese roll-up with Italian coleslaw baby carrots and sugar-free Jell-O

Post-Lunch Snack

Some light cheese wheels (try Mini Babybels just 1 - 2) with grape tomatoes Pre-Dinner Snack (can be skipped)

10 peanuts still in the shell (that's 20 individual nuts)

Dinner

Broccoli slaw and snow peas sautéed in a teaspoon of

peanut or canola oil with chicken and lettuce wraps and artificially sweetened sugar-free Jell-O

Day 12

Breakfast

Lean roast beef (1 ounce) with scrambled eggs and low-sodium tomato juice (4 - 6 ounces)

Pre-Lunch Snack

Non-fat artificially sweetened light yogurt (4 ounces) with 10 cashews

Lunch

Ham and Swiss roll-ups (2 - 3) with Italian coleslaw cucumbers (sliced) and artificially sweetened sugar-free Jell-O

Post-Lunch Snack

Celery sticks with light string cheese sticks (1 - 2) Pre-Dinner Snack (can be skipped)

¼ cup of guacamole with pepper strips

Dinner

Grilled fresh asparagus salad with grilled steak and sugar-free artificially sweetened Jell-O

Day 13

Breakfast

An omelet with diet cranberry juice (4 - 6 ounces)

Pre-Lunch Snack

Light cheese wedges (1 - 2) with some baby carrots Lunch

A large cheeseburger (no buns!) with a side salad and some sugar-free artificially sweetened Jell-O

Post-Lunch Snack

Non-fat artificially sweetened light yogurt with 20 walnuts Pre-Dinner Snack (can be skipped)

Swiss cheese (1 - 2 slices only made from 2% milk) with 10 cashews Dinner

Green beans with tomatoes (sliced) along with coleslaw or a side salad; sloppy joes (again no buns!) and sugar-free artificially sweetened Jell-O

Day 14

Breakfast

Boiled eggs (1 - 2) with some bacon along with low-sodium tomato juice (4 - 6 ounces)

Pre-Lunch Snack

Light yogurt (4 ounces) with 10 walnuts

Lunch

Sliced tomatoes with baby carrots a side salad with Italian or oil and vinegar based dressing some grilled chicken breast and sugar-free artificially sweetened Jell-O

Post-Lunch Snack

Grape tomatoes with light string cheese sticks (1 - 2) Pre-Dinner Snack (can be skipped)

10 peanuts still in the shell (20 single peanuts)

Dinner

A chicken salad (made of tomatoes, sliced scallions, sliced avocado or guacamole black beans, sliced pepper, lettuce, grilled chicken with 2 teaspoons of light-shredded cheese and ranch dressing) along with sugar-free artificially sweetened Jell-O

Chapter Four DASH Diet: Second Gear

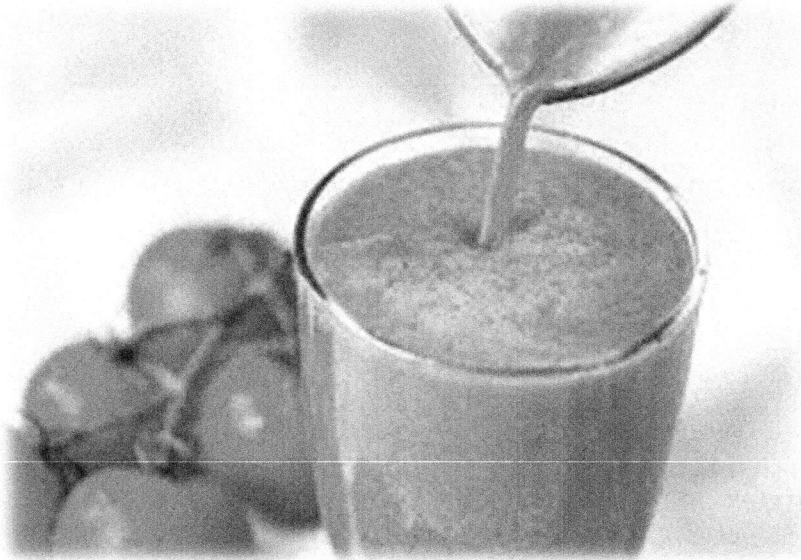

Well, look at you! You've conquered the first two weeks of the DASH diet. I'm giving you a standing ovation. If you followed this faithfully, I'm certain your clothes don't quite fit anymore because your stomach is smaller and your waist is leaner.

I'm pretty certain at this point you're bored of all the eggs and the Jell-O, and you just want some good old fashioned fruit in your mouth. Patience Padawan. We're going to fix that in stage two.

Excited? Good.

You're still going to eat all the DASH foods, but in this stage, we're going to add in some fruits, wholegrain, and more dairy and/or dairy substitutes. You're going to find this second stage a lot easier than the first because you've already got a solid foundation to work with. You've made eating healthy - the DASH way - into a habit. So let's kick things up a notch.

DASH Approved Foods for Stage 2

So we're ready to burn some more fat. Here's a simple list of foods which will be a part of your diet during

Stage 2.

Foods for Every Day

High-protein low-fat foods like fish, poultry, lean meats, eggs, beans lentils, and soy foods (2 - 3 servings)

Non-starchy veggies, peas, and corn (4 servings or more) Seeds and nuts (1 - 2 servings)

Wholegrain (Optional. No more than 1 - 2 servings) Non-fat or low-fat dairy - cheese yogurt and milk (3 - 4 servings) Note: You'll be having protein with each meal and each snack Foods for Once-In-A-While

Refined sugary or starchy foods (3 - 4 servings per week) To be clear, this could be the equivalent of a smaller than usual portion of dessert or bread if you're dining out. It could also be 2 slices of pizza in a month. Tempted to have much more than that? Fill your belly up with some salad.

Why encourage some starchy and sugary foods in this stage? The idea is you're not going to feel like you're depriving yourself of some carb-loaded goodness. However, you want to make sure you save your allotted carb quota for something that's real y delicious. Something you won't regret eating. However, you should consider staying away from pasta and low-carb bread. If you're going to have carbs make it unique. I don't know about you, but pizza always has a place in my heart.

Other Foods

You're going to have these in moderate amounts okay? Don't go overboard.

High-protein low saturated fat foods

Lentils soy soy-based foods and beans

Non-fat or low-fat cheeses

Fish, poultry, and lean meats

Whole eggs, egg whites or egg substitutes

Non-fat milk

Yogurt. Your yogurt should have no added sugar or at the very worst a negligible amount of sugar. Also for a 6-ounce serving, you want it less than 100 calories.

Opting for an 8-ounce serving? Then go for one that's no more than 120 calories.

Nuts and seeds

Fatty fish

Heart-friendly fats

Olives avocados

Vegetable oils, particularly nut oils, canola oil, and olive oil. No coconut oil or palm oil allowed.

Why? They've got high levels of saturated fat.

Oil-based salad dressings. It goes without saying that the dressings should be made using only the oils we listed above. A wee bit of mayonnaise is also allowed.

Foods to indulge in

You can have as much sugar-free Jell-O as you want. No limits. You can also enjoy as much as veggies as you like as long as they're non-starchy. Definitely stay away from winter squash corn and potatoes. If you absolutely insist on having some corn don't overindulge.

Foods to keep a lid on

Other than beans, you must limit your intake of starchy foods and sugary foods. So limit your pasta, potatoes, bread and other foods like that. You can also have some ketchup and barbeque sauce.

Stay away from food fried in batter. Also, you may not have pretzels rice cakes and other similar foods. Don't have foods which are way too high in saturated fats as well as hydrogenated or trans fats. Pastries, crackers, and cookies would fall under this category. Also, limit your intake of reduced-sugar cookies and pastries. Better yet, don't touch them. Research shows once you cut down sugar, you begin to crave it less. Plus you're going to help your taste buds better appreciate taste without needed some help from sugar.

If you're going to have some caffeine make sure you take it along with a snack or a meal. Want some alcohol? Drink in moderation. If you can just avoid it altogether since alcohol is a wonderful nutritious source of empty calories. If you really can't forfeit alcohol then you may have some wine. No more than 3 ½ ounces. Also when having the wine note that you'll be forfeiting one serving of fruit.

One last thing: definitely don't have food that doesn't taste good to you. No matter what.

Helpful Tips for Stage Two of The DASH Diet

Get a lot of fluids. You'll need at least 8 glasses a day. Caffeinated drinks and Jell-O also count toward your recommended daily fluid intake.

Don't skip meals and don't skip snacks. Remember we need your blood sugar nice and even and we need to avoid getting so hungry you overeat.

You can workout for 30 minutes or more now. You could opt for some strength training which will help you build muscle which burns fat even when you're not active. You can also do some aerobics such as running, biking or even just walking (or power-walking). Why am I asking you to do more exercise now? Because in this second stage you'll find you have even more energy than before.

Really color your plate. Throw in all sorts of veggies.

Take measurements particularly of your waist. Anytime you notice it's growing wider again you can return to Stage One till you notice your waist circumference dropping.

Take pictures! You'll love what you see overtime and you'll be motivated to keep going!

Remember, eating healthy is a habit for you now. Tell yourself you can't help but eat healthily. When you constantly tell yourself with feeling "I only eat healthily; it just feels better" you'll be reinforcing that idea in your mind, and you're more likely to stay consistent.

Focus on your results, and keep the goal in sight! You've come so far. Too late to quit. Keep going!

DASH Diet Stage 2 Serving Sizes

This list is just to give you an idea of the serving sizes

you'll need when in this second stage.

Bear in mind that if you're a larger man, you'll need a larger serving of foods high in protein.

Fruits

¼ cup of dried fruit

½ cup of canned fruit

1 cup of diced fruit (raw)

4 ounces of juice (alternatively a small or medium-sized fruit Veggies)

½ cup of cooked veggies

1 cup of leafy veggies

6 ounces of veggie juice

Nuts Seeds Beans

¼ cup of nuts

¼ cup of seeds

¼ cup of beans

Dairy

½ ounce of cottage cheese

1 ounce of cheese

8 ounces of milk (alternatively 8 ounces of yogurt)
Fish, Poultry, Eggs, Lean Meats

3 - 5 ounces of fish

3 - 5 ounces of poultry

3 - 5 ounces of lean meats

Note that 3 ounces is the equivalent of a woman's palm; 4 ounces is the equivalent of a woman's palm and thumb; 5 ounces is roughly the same size as a man's palm Also note that 1 egg is 1 ounce of protein and 2 egg whites also equal 1 ounce.

Fats and Fatty Sauces

1 teaspoon of oil

1 teaspoon of butter

1 tablespoon of salad dressing

Grains Sugars and Starches

½ cup of pasta corn potatoes or cereal (oatmeal wheat or grits) ⅓ cup of rice

¼ of a bagel ½ of an English muffin or a hot dog or hamburger bun 1 slice of bread

1 ounce of dry cereal (keep it between 80 - 100 calories) 2 cups of popcorn

2 small -sized cookies

Stage Two Food Suggestions

Just like the food suggestions we gave for Stage One, we're going to have some suggestions for this second stage. Keep in mind that you can make it your own as always. Just be certain not to overindulge in grains. You want 3 servings of grains a day and no more than that. Also, you must get 2 - 3 servings of dairy, 5 servings of veggies, and at least 3 servings of fruit each day. No exceptions. Use this guide as you wish. Once you're done reading through if you have a problem figuring things out I've got some meal plans you can follow after this!

Breakfasts

High-Protein Breakfasts

Eggs or egg substitutes (you may sometimes use cheese for a day or two) Bacon or ham (1 - 2 slices) or soy options

Milk or yogurt

4 ounces of juice (optional)

Roll-ups can make a great substitute if you're not a fan of eggs.

Cereal Breakfasts

Whole grain cereal. This must have less than 5 grams of sugar per serving. A serving by weight is 1 ounce, and by volume, it's equal to ½ cup of oatmeal. It must be no more than 100 calories.

You may sweeten your cereal with fruit.

Yogurt milk or hot chocolate (made with skim milk cocoa powder and a sugar substitute) 4 ounces of juice

Pre-Lunch Snacks

Along with some protein, you may have no more than 2 servings of the following:

Vegetables (celery, sliced peppers, radishes, carrots, grape or cherry, tomatoes, and cucumbers)

Yogurt (4 - 6 ounces unsweetened or artificial y sweetened) 4 ounces of low-fat cheese

1 serving of fruit

¼ cup of nuts or even less. That's 20 nuts. Having cheese with your nuts? Then you only get 10 nuts.

Lunches

Chicken and/or tuna salad, egg salad, egg white salad

Alternatively veggie salad with some protein and dressing. No croutons. You may add regular cheese. Better if you choose light cheese.

Roll-ups of low-fat cheese ham lean roast beef or turkey Along with the above you may add:

1 serving of fruit

Yogurt (4 - 6 ounces unsweetened or artificial y sweetened) or milk (8 ounces) Side salad and/or veggies with dressing

Nuts (at least 10 at most 20)

Sugar-free Jell-O

Post-Lunch Snacks

In addition to the foods listed as pre-lunch snacks, you may add: Pepper strips dipped in ¼ cup of hummus, vegetable-oil based salad dressing (or Italian dressing) or guacamole

10 peanuts (20 single nuts) still in the shell.

You may add a pre-dinner snack if you like based on

these snacks. It's optional.

Dinners

Salad with Italian dressing or oil and balsamic dressing, Fish, poultry or lean meat

Non-starchy vegetables (with reduced-fat cheese if you like)

Milk (if you like)

Got a crazy pasta craving? You can have some meaty pasta sauce (or pasta sauce with beans) on your veggies. Add in some cheese broil it, and you're good to go. You also have the option of using spaghetti squash to replace the pasta.

Some no-crust pizza would make for a great dinner too.

Desserts

1 serving of fruit

Sugar-free Jell-O

Fudge bars with no added sugars. Must be less than 100 calories. You may not have desserts with high-fat or excess calories.

Dining Out?

You can still follow Stage Two of the DASH diet easily. Just remember to check out the restaurant's menu first before you step out the door!

Breakfasts

Bacon or other lean meat

Omelets, eggs, oatmeal, or a whole grain cereal of your choice. (Be sure to have no more than 1 serving)

1 serving of fruit and/or tomatoes

4 ounces of juice

Milk (8 ounces) or unsweetened yogurt (4 - 6 ounces) You may replace potatoes or toast with fruit and vegetable instead

Lunches

A burger without the bun or grilled chicken along with a side salad vegetables and/or some coleslaw

Any salad with a good high-protein food

Yogurt or skim milk

Dinners

Fish, poultry or lean meat

Side veggies

Side salad with Italian dressing, oil-based dressing, or balsamic dressing. You may have a very very small amount of desert. Make sure it's really good stuff and check with yourself to see if you're still hungry or simply channeling your inner Oliver Twist.

When Grocery Shopping for Stage Two...

Make sure you stock up on the following:

Eggs

Egg substitutes (you may choose the ones with vegetables or without.) Sugar-free Jell-O

Skim milk

Individually packaged light cheeses, light string cheese, light cottage cheese (get the 4-ounce size)

Lean deli meats

Fish, poultry, and lean meats. Make sure to get the leanest meats you can. You can get beef tenderloin, pork tenderloin, sirloin all round cuts, chuck cuts and so on. You have lots of options to choose from.

Have fun!

Beans and soy or soy-based foods

Sliced light cheeses

Unsweetened or artificially sweetened non-fat yogurt. Be sure to also include 4-ounce sizes to serve as snacks. Also, remember there must be no more than

120 calories per 8-ounce yogurt and no more than 100 for 6 ounces.

Fresh fruits and veggies

Vegetable oils such as canola oil, olive oil, and nut oil, Salad dressings based on vegetable oils

Salads (tuna, chicken, egg, salads)

Nuts (preferably still in the shell). As with Stage One, my advice remains the same. Having to shell the nuts will slow down the rate at which you eat them, and you're more likely to get full on just a few than if you were able to scarf them down your mouth straight away.

Hummus

Guacamole

Now that you're done shopping for Stage Two of the DASH diet, I want you to refer back to that post-it note. Review the commitments you made to yourself.

When you followed Stage One of the DASH diet, were

there any challenges you faced that you had not seen crop up before? I want you to write them down. Next, think of effective creative ways you could deal with those challenges. Write them down and commit to following through.

Now one more thing. Take your before photo (from before you started the DASH diet) and take your after photo (after you completed Stage One of the DASH diet). Stick them both on the fridge right below the post-it note.

I can't wait till you post your third picture on the fridge and see just how far you've come!

Chapter Five DASH Diet Stage Two: Meal Plans

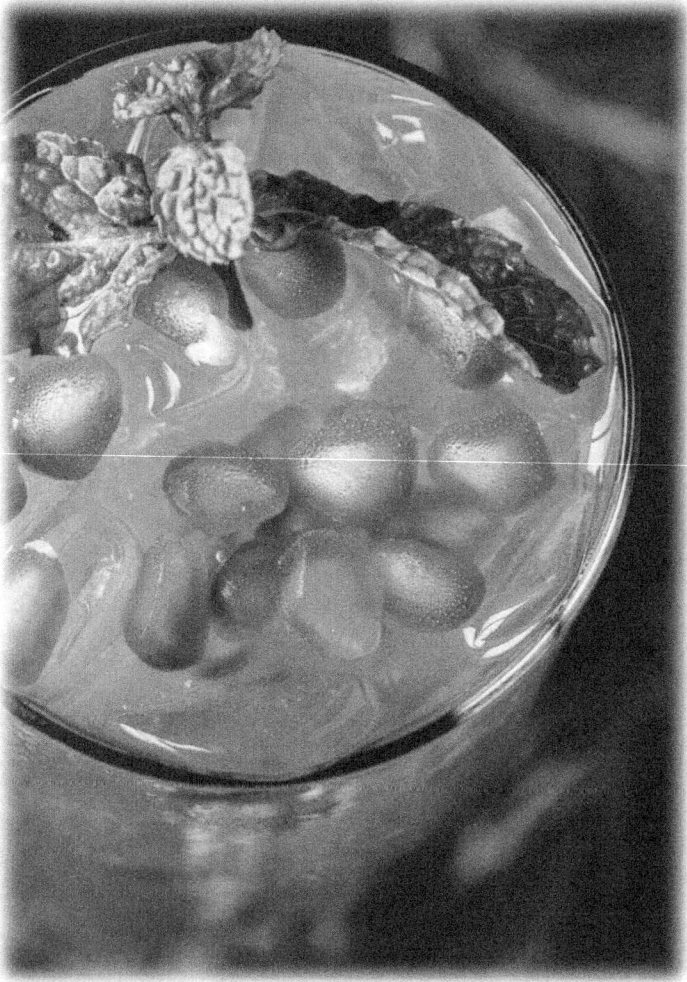

Now it's time for some all-new menus! I bet you're pretty stoked to be eating something new.

You've got more choices. Milk and fruit are back! As are your whole wheat bread and some cereals and some utterly delicious desserts.

Feel free to play with the menu. Swap snacks and meals. Do whatever. Just stick to the recommended daily servings and you'll do just fine.

You now have more options when it comes to your drinks. You can have hot cocoa milk and lattes in addition to your juices and good old water. You can have some alcohol - wine like we already mentioned - but just go easy, stick to the recommended daily serving size, and you won't pile the pounds back on. While you decide to have some wine, I implore you to consider skipping it altogether, so you don't get tempted to slide back into your old eating habits. Okay? Cool.

Meal Plan for DASH Diet Stage Two

Day 1

Breakfast

¾ cup or 1 ounce of low-sugar wheat cereal with skim milk (8 ounces) and raspberries or strawberries (4 - 6 ounces)

Pre-Lunch Snack (can be skipped)

1 to 2 wedges of light cheese with grape tomatoes Lunch

Baby carrots with a small plum and 2 or 3 turkey and Swiss roll-ups Post-Lunch Snack

Light yogurt (6 ounces) with 10 cashews.

Pre-Dinner Snack (can be skipped)

20 individual peanuts still in the shell

Dinner

Fresh asparagus with tilapia (pan-seared or grilled with 1 tablespoon of olive oil and some butter); some mango-melon salsa and sugar-free artificially sweetened Jell-O

Day 2

Breakfast

Boiled eggs (1 or 2) with hot cocoa (make it with 1 heaped spoon of unsweetened cocoa 8 ounces of skim milk and 2 packs of Truvia or Splenda); light cranberry juice (6 - 8 ounces); and strawberries (4 - 6 ounces).

Note: Light cranberry juice is tastier than diet cranberry juice; however, it does have more calories as well.

Pre-Lunch Snack (can be skipped)

Light yogurt (6 ounces non-fat artificially sweetened) with 10 ounces of almonds Lunch

Pepper strips with a side salad or some coleslaw; a turkey and Swiss sandwich (with a slice of non-fat Swiss cheese, your preferred veggies, and condiments on some whole wheat bread); and some sugar-free artificially sweetened Jell-O

Post-Lunch Snack

1 to 2 wedges of light cheese with 1 Clementine orange Pre-Dinner Snack (can be skipped)

Pepper strips with ¼ to ½ a cup of guacamole or hummus Dinner

Meaty sauce over some spaghetti squash along with a side salad (Italian vinaigrette oil and vinegar or balsamic dressing) and a fudge bar with no added sugar

Day 3

Breakfast

½ a banana (could be medium or large) with ½ a cup of cooked oatmeal (throw in some Splenda or Truvia some chopped nuts of your choice and some cinnamon if you like); low-sodium tomato juice (4 - 6 ounces) and a latte (use 2 ounces of espresso and 8 ounces of skim milk)

Pre-Lunch Snack (can be skipped)

Some baby carrots with a stick of light cheese

Lunch

Sliced bell peppers with a tuna salad ½ a pita pocket (must be whole wheat) with some veggies of your choice and some sugar-free artificially sweetened Jell-O

Post-Lunch Snack

10 cashews with strawberries (4 - 6 ounces)

Pre-Dinner Snack (can be skipped)

10 peanuts still in the shell

Dinner

Some green beans, tomatoes (sliced), a side salad with dressing of your choice. Some baked chicken, piccata, and raspberries (4 - 6 ounces) in 1 cup of non-fat artificially sweetened frozen yogurt

Day 4

Breakfast

A slice of toast (whole wheat) with 1 tablespoon of jam or jelly no more than 3 eggs (scrambled) some orange juice (4 - 6 ounces) and a latte or some skim milk (8 ounces only) Pre-Lunch Snack (can be skipped)

10 almonds with 4 - 6 ounces of blueberries

Lunch

Some Italian coleslaw 3 roast beef and cheese roll-ups with some veggies and a peach Post-Lunch Snack.

Light non-fat yogurt (artificially sweetened)

Pre-Dinner Snack (can be skipped)

Peanut butter (no more than 2 tablespoons please) and some baby carrots

Dinner

A side salad with some cheese and dressing of your choice combined with some zucchini lasagna and a fudge bar with no added sugar.

Day 5

Breakfast

Skim milk (8 ounces) with 1 heaped spoon of cocoa (unsweetened) and 2 packs of Truvia or Splenda for a cup of hot cocoa; 1 cup of raisin bran with some skim milk (4 ounces) and some orange juice or tangerine juice or any kind of juice with high potassium levels.

Pre-Lunch Snack (can be skipped)

Non-fat artificially sweetened light yogurt

Lunch

A whole wheat peanut butter and jelly sandwich. (Make sure your peanut butter is all-natural) some baby carrots, an apple (medium sized) and if you like a side salad with some Italian or vinaigrette dressing

Post-Lunch Snack

Some grape tomatoes along with 1 or 2 light string cheese sticks

Pre-Dinner Snack (can be skipped)

¼ cup of hummus or guacamole with some raw vegetables of your choice

Dinner

Some grilled chicken with ⅓ of a cup of brown rice and

a colorful salad plate with Italian or vinegar or oil-and-vinegar dressing along with some sugar-free artificially sweetened Jell-O

Day 6

Breakfast

Egg and vegetable omelet (1 - 3 eggs) with some Canadian bacon (2 - 3 slices) a latte (8 - 12 ounces) and some low-sodium tomato juice (4 -6 ounces)

Pre-Lunch Snack (can be skipped)

10 cashews with 4 - 6 ounces of strawberries

Lunch

A cheeseburger (buns must be whole wheat; if not go bunless); some broccoli coleslaw and a pear (small or medium)

Post-Lunch Snack

A plum with 1 or 2 deviled eggs

Pre-Dinner Snack (can be skipped)

20 single peanuts (still in the shell)

Dinner

Chicken salad topped with berries of your choice with a fudge bar (remember no added sugar)

Day 7

Breakfast

½ a banana, ¾ a cup of Grape, Nut Flakes, some skim milk (8 ounces) and some orange juice (4 - 6 ounces)

Pre-Lunch Snack (can be skipped)

1 to 2 wedges of light cheese with some baby carrots
Lunch

Some sliced cucumbers and tomatoes with some Italian coleslaw 1 or 2 vegetarian hot dogs (with whole wheat bread or tortilla along with your preferred condiments) and a sugar-free Jell-O cup

Post-Lunch Snack

10 almonds with some non-fat artificially sweetened light yogurt

Pre-Dinner Snack (can be skipped)

¼ of a cup to ½ a cup of hummus and some raw veggies

Dinner

A side salad with some oil and vinegar Italian or balsamic dressing along with some roasted chicken and veggies salad; some raspberries (4 - 6 ounces) in

1 cup of nonfat artificial y sweetened frozen yogurt

Day 8

Breakfast

1 blueberry waffle (whole-grain) with some blueberry jelly or jam boiled eggs (1 or 2) and hot chocolate DASH-style.

Pre-Lunch Snack (can be skipped)

10 walnuts with some non-fat artificially sweetened light yogurt Lunch.

Some sesame chicken salad along with 1 or 1 ½ cups cherries.

Post-Lunch Snack

2 tablespoons of peanut butter and some baby carrots or cucumbers

Pre-Dinner Snack (can be skipped)

6 low-sodium water crackers along with 1 slice of Swiss cheese (from 2% milk)

Dinner

A side salad along with some chicken frittata and a fudge bar with no added sugar

Day 9

Breakfast

A latte (8 - 12 ounces) with ½ of a medium banana, ½ a cup of cooked oatmeal (you may add some cinnamon and Splenda or Truvia or an artificial sweetener of your choice) and some light cranberry juice (4 - 6 ounces)

Pre-Lunch Snack (can be skipped)

Baby carrots with nonfat artificially sweetened yogurt

Lunch

Chicken and/or tuna salad in ½ a whole grain pit with vegetables of your choice some cucumber slices, a side salad with some Italian or vinaigrette dressing and a medium-sized plum

Post-Lunch Snack

Some cherry or grape tomatoes with some string cheese (1 or 2 sticks)

Pre-Dinner (can be skipped)

Some creamy cauliflower, mashed potatoes, ½ a cup of sweet corn, and meatloaf with a tablespoon of BBQ sauce or catsup if you like

Day 10

Breakfast

Boiled eggs (1 or 2) with strawberries (4 to 6 ounces) 8 to 12 ounces of hot cocoa and 4 to 6 ounces of orange juice or orange-tangerine juice

Pre-Lunch Snack (can be skipped)

1 to 2 wedges of light cheese with some cherry tomatoes or grape tomatoes Lunch.

Whole wheat bread with some Swiss and ham tomatoes and other veggies along with some Italian coleslaw or a side salad dressed with Italian dressing or vegetable oil-based dressing.

Finish off with 2 slices of fresh pineapple.

Post-Lunch Snack

10 almonds with 6 ounces of non-fat artificially sweetened light yogurt

Pre-Dinner Snack (can be skipped)

¼ cup of hummus or guacamole with raw veggies (or pepper strips)

Dinner

Some roasted Brussels sprouts with balsamic or vinaigrette dressing some salsa grilled pork loin and a fudge bar with no added sugar.

Day 11

Breakfast

Skim milk (8 ounces) with 1 shredded wheat biscuit strawberries (4 to 6 ounces) and some orange juice (4 to 6 ounces)

Pre-Lunch Snack (can be skipped)

Baby carrots or celery with a non-fat artificially sweetened light yogurt

Lunch

Poached chicken salad with some grapes and walnuts

Post-Lunch Snack

10 cashes with a medium plum or peach

Pre-Dinner Snack (can be skipped)

Swiss cheese from 2% milk (1 or 2 slices)

Dinner

Glazed carrots with a side salad and dressing of your choice grilled salmon and some raspberries (4 to 6 ounces) in non-fat artificially sweetened frozen yogurt

Day 12

Breakfast

An omelet (1 to 3 eggs) with a slice of toast (whole wheat) spread with jelly or jam; a cantaloupe wedge and some orange juice (4 to 6 ounces)

Pre-Lunch Snack (can be skipped)

1 to 2 wedges of light cheese with cherry tomatoes

Lunch

Some low-sodium tomato soup (4 ounces) with a chicken and/or tuna sandwich (use whole wheat bread and add in some lettuce some light cheese and any other veggies you prefer); some sliced rashes and an apple (small)

Post-Lunch Snack

10 cashews with a non-fat artificially sweetened light yogurt

Pre-Dinner Snack (can be skipped)

¼ to ½ a cup of guacamole with pepper strips

Dinner

1 cup of petite sweet peas with blackened chicken with avocado-papaya salsa, a side salad or some coleslaw with your preferred dressing and some strawberries (about 4 to 6 ounces) in a cup of non-fat artificially sweetened frozen yogurt.

Day 13

Breakfast

½ of a medium-sized banana (sliced) with 1 cup of wheat cereal (with no added sugar) and some skim milk (8 ounces). End with 4 - 6 ounces of orange juice.

Pre-Lunch Snack (can be skipped)

10 walnuts with some non-fat artificially sweetened light yogurt Lunch.

Turkey roll-ups with some raspberry salsa (1 or 2) with a side salad and your favorite dressing.

Wrap up with 1 Clementine orange

Post-Lunch Snack

Celery sticks with some light string cheese sticks (1 or 2) Pre-Dinner Snack (can be skipped)

20 single peanuts still in their shells

Dinner

Some roasted broccoli, carrots, and cauliflower with some broiled halibut; a blood orange lettuce and romaine salad with a fudge bar (no added sugar).

Day 14

Breakfast

Boiled eggs (1 or 2) with ½ of an English muffin (made from whole grain) with some butter or margarine on top; some late (8 to 12 ounces), some strawberries (4 to 6 ounces) and some low-sodium tomato juice (4 to 6 ounces)

Pre-Lunch Snack (can be skipped)

Cherry tomatoes with some light string cheese sticks

Lunch

Cucumber and tomato slices with some Italian

coleslaw or a side salad (with your preferred dressing) and a grilled chicken sandwich (use whole wheat).

Finish with a plum peach or pear.

Post-Lunch Snack

20 single peanuts with 6 ounces of some non-fat artificially sweetened light yogurt

Pre-Dinner Snack (can be skipped)

Some pepper strips with hummus or guacamole or black bean salsa

Dinner

Mashed sweet potatoes with seasonings of your choice some meatloaf with catsup or BBQ sauce, green beans, and sliced peppers. Finish with 4 to 6 ounces of strawberries blueberries and raspberries.

Chapter Six Move Your Body

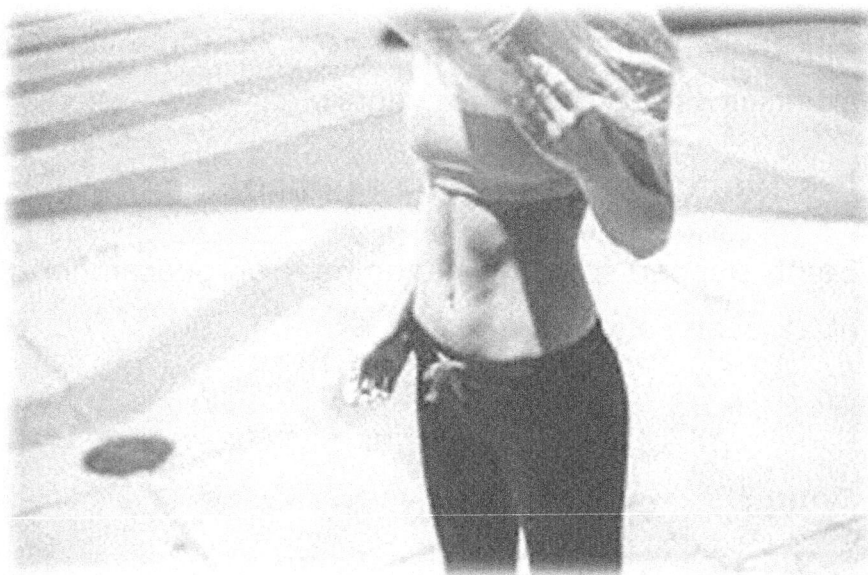

If you've been researching weight loss methods long enough, then you already know the basics of managing your weight. You have to keep a balance between the number of calories you consume (as in the amount of food you eat) and the number of calories you expend (as in the number of calories you lose when you're physical y active).

So we've already covered the calories you should be consuming in Stage One and Stage Two of the DASH diet. It's time to turn our attention to that fabulous amazing work of biological engineering called your "body."

Why Exercise Matters

When you consciously decide to do more physical activity than usual, it isn't because you're a masochist (at least I would hope not.) You understand how important it is to be physically active.

However, I'm going to list some reasons why exercise matters anyway. It's one thing to know it matters "somewhere in the back of my mind." It's another thing to have the reasons you should work out front and center as you embark on your weight loss journey with DASH. So here's why you should move your body more:

You'll fire up your metabolism.

Muscles burn fat. One great way to increase the amount of muscle in your body is to work out - particularly strength training. The more muscle you have then, the more efficient your metabolism will be because your muscles will burn fat even when you are at rest! So yes, you should workout and do so as often as you can manage. When you also consider the fact that as you age, you lose a fair bit of your muscle mass, you won't need to be told twice not to skip the gym. See as you get older you have less muscle. Less muscle means a slower metabolism. A slower metabolism means "Hello Beer Gut, my old friend." You definitely don't want that. Working out or engaging in more physical activity is a surefire way to avoid muscle loss and fat gain that comes with age. Plus don't you just love the idea of burning fat even when you're doing nothing? I do. So get your workout in.

You'll get stronger. Once upon a time, I used to be a couch potato. I was the couchiest potato that ever couch potatoed. That's how inactive I was. I packed on the pounds, and I got miserable. Once I decided something had to change. I set to cleaning up my diet and getting my workouts in. I lost the great weight. You know what is even more awesome? The incredible amount of strength that I've gained from working out! It's such a boost in confidence.

Besides being able to beat all my brothers at arm wrestling, getting a workout in makes it easier for you to do your usual day-to-day activities. Also, you're less likely to suffer from injuries in the process.

You'll be healthier. It's great to be fit lean and sexy and all. However, exercise is much more than weight loss. Even if you're not dropping much weight, you'll find that exercise has immense health benefits. You have less risk of getting diabetes, some cancers, heart diseases, and strokes. When you work out, you're more likely to live long. Your mood gets a marvelous boost.

Also, your libido will thank you. Think I'm lying? Why

don't you start working out and see for yourself?

If these reasons have motivated you to want to be more active, then congratulations! Wondering where to begin? You can start easy. Don't worry, you don't have to go deadlift 500 pounds in the gym on your first day. I want you fit and healthy, not disabled.

A caveat: before you take any advice in this book regarding exercise, please consult with your doctor, okay? Especially if you have certain medical issues which might be aggravated by physical activity.

Walk The Pounds Away

When you first start working out, you want to begin as easy as possible. If you've always been inactive and then you suddenly decide "Hey I want to do Insanity Max 30 or P90X" well you're asking for a whole world of hurt. You're less likely to succeed because you'll find yourself avoiding pain. See unless you're some type of masochist, you're naturally wired to seek pleasure and avoid pain. So how do we exploit this? What kind of workout would be best to inspire you to continue while giving you sure safe results?

One word: walking.

If you've been a lifelong couch potato, haven't worked out in a long time - if ever - I highly suggest you start off with walking. It's a great way to melt the pounds away. Why? You can think of it wherever and whenever you want. You don't need workout equipment. You don't need a gym membership. It won't cost you anything - except for calories which I'm sure you're more than happy to lose!

Before You Walk

You have to get the perfect pair of shoes for walking. There are shoes specially designed for taking walks, so get those. If you can't go for some running shoes. Make sure they're a really good pair, and they fit just right. Cross trainers are pretty good too. While you're at it, invest in new socks - unless you want blisters on your feet.

Buying new shoes? Don't take them for your walk immediately. Take some time to break them in. Wear them about at home.

Figure out the route you'll be taking. You don't want

to waste moments during your walk, trying to figure out where to head next. So decide on your routes and follow those.

Create set dates and times to walk. With some structure, it's easier to commit, and you give yourself no excuses to postpone your walks.

If it's cold outside, dress appropriately. However, make sure whatever you're wearing, you can take off a piece of clothing or more as you get warmer during your walk.

Is the weather horrible? Perhaps some heavy rain or snow? Then you can take a walk around the mall. There are some malls with mall-walking programs, so perhaps you could sign yourself up. Don't like the mall? Fine. Walk around your home or even on a spot. Be sure you're doing something interesting as you walk since there won't be much to look at in your home. You could try listening to an audiobook or watching your favorite TV show. There are also walking workout programs that you can try out. I highly recommend checking out Leslie Sansone's walking workouts. The best part about them is she's split them up into miles so you can hit your target easily without needing to look at your watch.

Rope in a friend. If you're walking with a friend, it makes it easier for you to commit to your walking program not to mention less boring. So find a friend who'll love to get fit too and walk together!

Another thing: don't go in hard and fast. Doing more than you can handle is a surefire way to make yourself give up. Take it easy. Just show up and do what you can.

Note that the faster you walk, the more you burn per mile. Also, the heavier you are, the more calories you'll burn.

Finally, keep a record of your walking workouts. It's nice when you look back and see the miles add up.

Walking Regimens You Can Follow

Beginner regimen

If you're very heavy, completely unfit or quite old, then this is a great walking regimen for you to follow.

Distance

Time

Frequency (Per Week)

1st Week

¼ of a mile

10 to 15 minutes

2 to 3 times

2nd Week

½ of a mile

12 to 15 minutes

2 to 3 times

3rd Week

¾ of a mile to 1 mile

20 to 25 minutes

3 times

4th Week

¾ of a mile to 1 mile

20 to 25 minutes

3 times

5th Week

1 mile to 1 ½ mile

20 to 30 minutes

3 to 4 times

6th Week

1 mile to 1 ½ mile

20 to 30 minutes

3 to 4 times

7th Week

1 ½ mile to 2 miles

27 to 36 minutes

3 to 4 times

8th Week

1 ½ mile to 2 miles

27 to 36 minutes

3 to 4 times

9th Week

2 miles to 2 ½ miles

35 minutes to 44 minutes

4 times

10th Week

2 miles to 2 ½ miles

35 minutes to 44 minutes

4 times

11th Week

2 ½ miles to 3 miles

43 minutes to 51 minutes

4 times

12th Week

2 ½ miles to 3 miles

43 minutes to 51 minutes

4 times

13th Week

2 ½ miles to 3 miles

40 minutes to 48 minutes

4 times

14th Week

2 ½ miles to 3 miles

40 minutes to 48 minutes

4 times

15th Week

3 miles to 3 ½ miles

48 minutes to 56 minutes

4 to 5 times

Moderate regimen

Having completed that regimen, you can move on to this next one when you're ready. If you're already somewhat fit, forget the beginner regimen and start with this one.

Distance

Time

Frequency (Per Week)

1st Week

½ a mile to 1-mile minutes

8 minutes to 15

2 to 3 times

2nd Week

1 ½ mile

23 minutes

2 to 3 times

3rd Week

1 ½ mile to 2 miles

21 minutes to 26 minutes

3 times

4th Week

1 ½ mile to 2 miles

21 minutes to 26 minutes

3 times

5th Week

2 miles to 2 ½ miles

29 minutes to 39 minutes

3 to 4 times

6th Week

2 miles to 2 ½ miles

29 minutes to 39 minutes

3 to 4 times

7th Week

2 ½ miles to 3 miles

35 minutes to 42 minutes

3 to 4 times

8th Week

2 ½ miles to 3 miles

35 minutes to 42 minutes

3 to 4 times

9th Week

2 ½ miles to 3 miles

34 minutes to 41 minutes

3 to 4 times

10th Week

2 ½ miles to 3 miles

34 minutes to 41 minutes

3 to 4 times

11th Week

2 ½ miles to 3 miles

33 minutes to 39 minutes

4 times

12th Week

2 ½ miles to 3 miles

33 minutes to 39 minutes

4 times

13th Week

3 miles to 3 ½ miles

39 minutes to 46 minutes

4 to 5 times

14th Week

3 miles to 3 ½ miles

39 minutes to 46

4 to 5 times minutes

15th Week

3 ½ miles to 4 miles

46 minutes to 52 minutes

4 to 5 times

Advanced regimen

If you've successfully followed the previous regimen, then follow this advanced regimen. Fairly active? Then skip the previous two and do this.

Distance

Time

Frequency (Per Week)

1st Week

½ a mile to 1 mile

6 minutes to 12 minutes

2 to 3 times

2nd Week

1 ½ mile

18 minutes

2 to 3 times

3rd Week

1 ½ mile to 2 miles

18 minutes to 24 minutes

3 times

4th Week

1 ½ mile to 2 miles

18 minutes to 24 minutes

3 times

5th Week

2 miles to 2 ½ miles

24 minutes to 30 minutes

3 to 4 times

6th Week

2 miles to 2 ½ miles

24 minutes to 30 minutes

3 to 4 times

7th Week

2 ½ miles to 3 miles

30 minutes to 36 minutes

3 to 4 times

8th Week

2 ½ miles to 3 miles

30 minutes to 36 minutes

3 to 4 times

9th Week

3 miles to 3 ½ miles

36 minutes to 42 minutes

3 to 4 times

10th Week

3 miles to 3 ½ miles

36 minutes to 42 minutes

3 to 4 times

11th Week

3 miles to 3 ½ miles

33 minutes to 40 minutes

4 times

12th Week

3 miles to 3 ½ miles

33 minutes to 40 minutes

4 times

13th Week

3 ½ miles to 4 miles

42 minutes to 48 minutes

4 to 5 times

14th Week

3 ½ miles to 4 miles

42 minutes to 48 minutes

4 to 5 times

15th Week

3 ½ miles to 4 miles

40 minutes to 44 minutes

4 to 5 times

Revving Up Your Body's Engine

No doubt you already know there are lots of ways for you to get fit. Walking is one. Dancing is another. Lifting mighty forks of lasagna from your plate to your mouth is another as well. No, that last one isn't obviously.

If walking isn't for you or you've been walking and feel the need to do a lot more then it's time for a new program! How do you pick one that's right for you?

First, figure out where you'll rather work out. Will you go to a gym or stay at home? I prefer home workouts because as soon as I'm up, I change clothes and get started right away no excuses.

You might prefer the gym. There's no one right way to do this.

If you decide you'll be doing your exercise at home, you might need to invest in a good pair of dumbbells (you can get adjustable ones so you can add or decrease weight as required). You might also need a yoga mat some bands maybe a pull-up bar or a good old fashioned bike. Just figure out what you need. If you follow a home workout program, you should be given a list of the workout equipment which will be used. If you do decide to workout at home and you have no experience, please consider enlisting a personal trainer's services.

If you choose to be a gym rat awesome! There's lots of equipment to work with. Another great thing is that gyms offer classes of all sorts so you could choose to attend a spin class or a dance class or do some yoga. Whatever works for you. You can also take advantage of the personal trainers on hand at the gym who will figure out where you're at physically and work out a plan to help you achieve your fitness goals.

How to Make A Habit of Exercising

Make sure you love whatever you choose to do. No sense spending so much time and energy on something that makes you plain miserable.

Don't go overboard. Stick to a program that's great for your level of fitness.

Keep your goals as realistic as possible. You know what the big picture is. Chunk down the goals into smaller bits then crush them.

Give yourself some time. Your body will take a while before it gets used to your program.

Don't quit just because you didn't see results the first day or week or month. You didn't pack on the pounds in a day. They're not going to melt away in a day either.

Make sure you have rest days. Your body needs time

to recover as does your mind so you can get back at it the next session stronger and ready to roll.

Find a workout buddy. When you're going the journey with someone, it's easier to commit and follow through. Also, it's much more fun.

Don't push your body too hard. Listen to it. Stop if something doesn't feel right and get yourself checked out before you continue. There's the usual pain from working out, but there's the kind of pain where you know something's off. Don't push through that sort of pain.

Get some work in every day. It's better to do something than to do absolutely nothing. Don't beat yourself up about not getting in enough reps or sets. Just show up and be glad you did. Show up for yourself every day.

Building Muscle with Strength Training

Chances are you've heard over and over again if you want to lose weight then you're better off doing lots and lots of cardio. Cardio's great. I'm not going to knock it or anything. It's great for getting your heart beating and your lungs pumping and oh my does it burn a lot of calories!

However, something just as awesome as cardio (I'll say more awesome, but that's just me) is strength training. I am speaking not just based off of scientific facts but from personal experience as well.

I started off with cardio when I decided to resign from my position as Executive Couch Potato. I saw results, and I loved them. Then my buddy Marcus said to me one day, "James, why don't you try lifting?" I scoffed. I thought it was just overkill at the time. But then I thought about it, and I decided to give it a whirl for at least 1 month. I haven't looked back since then.

Why should you incorporate strength training along with the DASH diet? I've already mentioned before that the more muscle you have, the more fat you're going to burn even when you're not doing anything physically demanding. Strength training is the absolute best way to build lean muscle mass, which melts the fat away!

If you're a cardio lover, I can already hear you whining. Here's the thing though: when I took up strength training, my cardio got easier, and I suffered far lesser injuries too. This is not just something anecdotal; it's backed up by science. Don't believe me? Do a quick Google search.

Even better, why don't you try strength training yourself? The best way to really know is to have your own experience.

There's a lot to talk about when it comes to strength training, but this book is about the DASH diet and how to make it work even better for you. I can, however, help you out if you're trying to figure out how to take on strength training.

First of all, where do you love to work out? At the gym? At home? Can you afford the gym? Do you feel at ease working out in public? These are questions you need to ask yourself.

Next, you need to figure out how often you want to do strength training. For the best results, I'll advise you to do thirty minutes of strength training at least two times a week. Three times is better. You're going to see results faster. You want to make sure you've got a day or two in between your strength training sessions, so your muscles have time to rebuild and recover. On days you're not strength training you can get in your cardio whether it's High-Intensity Interval Training (HIIT) or Low-Intensity Steady State cardio (LISS). Whatever you do commit.

Consistency is key if you want massive results.

Wondering what workout programs to try? Do a quick Google search, and you should see a few good ones. Just be sure you have the equipment on hand if you're going to work out at home.

You could also check out Darebee.com. They've got amazingly easy to follow workout programs, and they're all for free!

If you're skeptical about whether you should be exercising since you think it would make you hungrier and therefore eat more here's the thing: you don't have to worry about that. Studies have shown you're less likely to get hungry after a workout session because working out will increase your body temperature. This consequently reduces your appetite.

Sure your body will reset to its usual temperature and then you'll want to eat; however, remember all those snacks we've included in the meal plan? Once you've faithfully planned your meals a head you'll be just fine. Reach for your DASH approved snack when the munchies hit.

Making Exercise Your Way of Life

Did you know there are tons of ways to make exercising a part of your everyday life? I mean without having to hit the gym or pop in a workout DVD. When you do chores, go biking, take a walk, go hiking with friends or play games with them, you're actually much better off than just parking your behind on a couch and watching reruns of Game of Thrones.

There's research that shows taking part in activities which get you moving is actually just as great as hitting the gym. This is a real study in the Journal of the American Medical Association. Apparently, all you need is an excuse to move for just 30 minutes every day, and you can get all the benefits you'd get from a proper workout.

Sadly people avoid moving. They avoid activity. Why walk 3 blocks when they can just drive?

Why take the stairs when the elevator's working fine? Does this sound like you? Then you need to start making some better choices if you value your health and your life.

What situations can you take advantage of to get moving? You could choose to get up and take quick brisk walks down the hallway at work every now and then. Need to meet with a colleague?

Do it while walking up and down the hallway. Don't send an email to your boss. Get up and head to her office instead. When you head to work, get off the bus, a couple of stops away and walk the rest of the way. Driving? Find a spot to park some distance away from work.

Lunchtime is a great time to get moving. So take a walk! When you're making phone calls get up pace stretch. Don't just sit there. On a work trip? Make sure you take advantage of the hotel's gym.

When at home you could take care of your yard yourself. All that weeding mowing (with a good old-fashioned push-mower) will surely help you burn some calories! Do chores at home yourself.

Got a dog? Start taking it out for walks. It will do you both some good. Need to hit the store? Try walking or riding a bike there. If you absolutely have to drive, you could park a good way away from the entrance.

Chapter Seven How to Set Goals and Crush Them

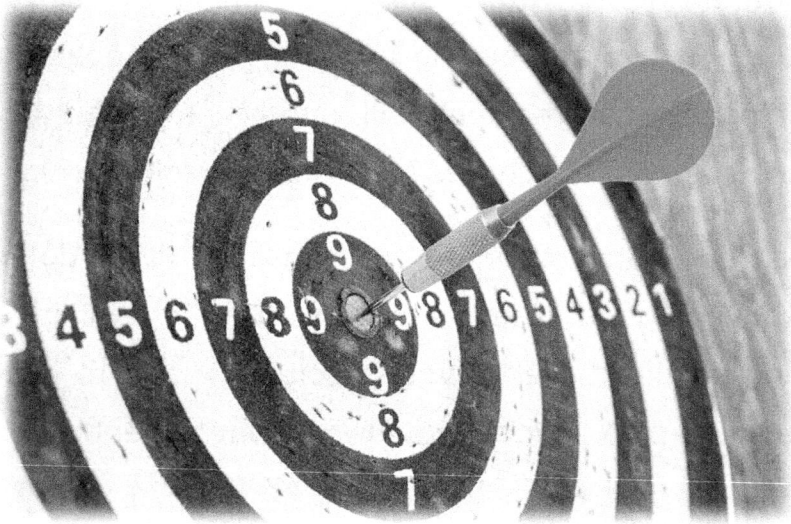

You now know how the DASH diet works. You understand how important it is to get some exercise in once you've transitioned from Stage One to Stage Two. Now how do we make sure you actually achieve your goals? How can you stay on target and hit your ideal weight? Beyond losing the weight, how do you make sure that you maintain your new weight?

To keep you on target we'll need to pay special attention to the steps you'll take to help you reach your goal weight and manage your weight better for life. See a great way to set yourself up for failure is to set goals that are unachievable and utterly unrealistic. Set goals up this way and you're going to fail successfully, my friend. I assume that's not what you want.

What's the better option then? You want goals that can be reached. You want realistic goals. Goals that put you on the path to success. Have you ever heard about SMART goals?

S - Specific

M - Measurable

A - Action-Oriented

R - Realistic

T - Timed

The thing is once your goals are SMART, you are more likely to make them happen. To tell the difference between SMART goals and non-SMART goals, I'm going to give you a couple of examples.

Say you declare to yourself, "I'm never having ice cream again till the day I die." Is this a SMART goal? No. It's noble at best, but it's really neither SMART nor smart (pun intended). "Till the day I die" is really not that specific because when will you die anyway? The time frame is so not specific. You can't measure it. You're not taking action. You've only said you "will not" have ice-cream again. That's not action. What will you do? That's action. It's not realistic because how do you go from regularly eating ice cream to just stopping cold turkey? Don't get me wrong - some people are great at quitting things cold turkey. Are you one of them? If not, how do you expect to achieve this goal?

A smarter version of this goal could be "I'm going to eat half the usual amount of ice cream I have just once a week." Much better.

Here's another goal: "I'm going to work out more." Again noble. Just not very SMART. Here's something better: "This week every time I come home from work, I'm going to strength train for 30 minutes before I shower and have dinner." Let's analyze this.

It's Specific because you said you'll "strength train" versus something more generic like "I'll exercise."

It's Measurable because you've said you'll do it for 30 minutes and you'll do it after work each day. If you go to work 5 times a week that's 5 times, you'll be working out.

It's Action-oriented because you've specifically mentioned something you will do, not what you won't do, or what you will stop doing. Get the difference?

It's Realistic because you can get in a 30-minute strength training session after work. This is easier to do than say a 2-hour workout. Good luck with that.

It's Timed since you've pegged this week as when

you'll choose to workout.

Why You Need to Be A Realist

Look I'm the dreamiest dreamer you'll ever know. However, I've had to learn from experience the importance of being a realist. What can I say? It's a balancing act.

See when you think about making a change - especially one that's so drastic - it's easy to feel like it's all just too much for you to handle. You feel overwhelmed. You don't think there's any point in trying since in your mind you've already failed. Can you imagine what it must be like being David having to face Goliath? That feeling applies when you take on gargantuan goals.

How do you fix this?

You do this by chunking down your goals. You make them as small as you can. Cut them up into smaller manageable pieces. Cut your goals in half and then maybe half of half. Does that sound like cheating? Does that sound like you wouldn't be achieving much if you did that? Well not true at all.

Let me give you two different scenarios here. In Scenario A, you've got a goal to lose 10 pounds in 2 weeks. You do everything you can to hit that goal. By the end of 2 weeks, you weigh yourself and... You've only lost 7 pounds! You start to think of all the effort, blood sweat, and tears you put into make this goal happen. You gave it your all and yet you failed. This failure weighs on you, undermines your confidence. You decide meh you're done. Why bother. Pfft. I'm just going to enjoy this here extra-large pizza all by myself.

Now let's look at Scenario B. You want to lose 10 pounds in 2 weeks. You decide yes that's what you'll like to do, but perhaps you should aim for something smaller. You decide you're going to lose 5 pounds in 2 weeks. By the end of your time limit, you weigh yourself and... Holy crapoly! You've not just lost 5 pounds you lost 2 more on top of that! You didn't just set a goal and hit it. You crushed it! How does that

149

feel? How do you feel? Amazing right? Perhaps even inspired to set another small goal and crush it!

Setting small goals allows them to not just be easily achievable but easy to surpass as well.

Even if you had lost exactly 5 pounds, guess what? You'll still feel great about it. You'll have the confidence to set another goal. You'll have the conviction that you can achieve it. Want in on a secret? That confidence in yourself spills over to other aspects of your life!

You want to be more social? Thinking of making 5 phone calls a day? How about just one a day? There. Nailed it. You want to write a book of about 25000 words? Thinking of writing 5000 words a day? Why don't you chunk it down to 2500 words a day? Or even just 500 a day if you don't have a time limit? There. Crushed it. If you remember nothing else about goals, remember this: set them small and you'll crush them hard.

In the beginning, it might feel like you're not doing much. But trust me those series of "little" actions you take toward your goals will snowball into something that will knock your socks off - in a good way. I should know. How do you think I set about writing this book? Small goals.

Crushed them. Next!

Focus on Today

What if you only had to follow your goal just for today? Wouldn't it feel easier to achieve? So you get through the day having accomplished your goal. You let tomorrow worry about itself. When tomorrow becomes another today all you have to do is focus on today again. That's it. Wash rinse repeat.

Next thing you know you've got a whole string of "today's" where you crushed your goal. Next thing you know, it becomes a habit. You don't even have to think about it. You find it just happens. If something happens to interrupt your routine or change your day you find yourself antsy itching to go get a "fix."

Do you have any idea how awesome it is when you've got a good addiction that's in line with your goals, and you're just constantly craving another fix? Also, success is addictive. Focusing on just today means you're more likely to succeed. You'll be looking forward to tomorrow's fix. Heck, you might find yourself doing a little something extra each day since you've knocked the day's goal out the park.

When you're planning your DASH meals or doing your workouts, just keep this at the back of your mind: "One day at a time." You can take the tip from the previous section and chunk it down even further. For your DASH diet meals focus on one meal at a time. If you've chosen walking as a way to get your exercise, think "one step at a time." Are you strength training?

Think "one rep at a time." You get the idea. Do this, and you'll succeed every time. I guarantee it.

If you don't. Feel free to print this book out and set it on fire while laying a curse on me.

Give Yourself A Pat On The Back

Another great way to ensure your continued success with your weight loss goals is to reward yourself each time you reach a goal. You ever heard of Pavlov's dog?

In the 1890s there was this guy named Ivan Pavlov. He was a Russian scientist. At the time he was researching dogs and their response to food. He set up a metronome within the dogs' hearing. He got no response from them toward it.

After this, Pavlov would get the metronome going right before he fed the dogs. He did this over and over again. After a while, he went back to just set up the metronome without feeding the dogs. What did he find? The dogs now reacted to the metronome by salivating.

What does this mean? You're not a dog after all. Let me break it down. If each time you successfully complete a goal you give yourself a reward after a while you'll find yourself automatically wanting to complete your goals since you've learned to associate completed goals with rewards.

For instance, if you decided that rather than snack on cotton candy you'll have celery sticks dipped in some delicious guacamole you can reward yourself for following through on that decision. Obviously, your reward should not be food-related. You could decide to buy yourself that new hat you've been wanting. You could decide you deserve to go see a movie or buy yourself a certain book you've been meaning to read.

Even better when you set your goals, incorporate the reward into them. Here's a good example:

"If I strength train after work for five days this week I'm going to get myself a nice new hair cut (or hair-do). Whatever your goals you absolutely must celebrate them when you've successfully accomplished them. You'll celebrate a loved one or a friend if something great happened to them, wouldn't you? So why not celebrate your accomplishments as well?

When it comes to rewards, you need to remember this one very important thing: Reward yourself for your behavior and not for your results. Rather than reward yourself for losing 10 pounds, reward yourself for taking the actions you had to in order to lose the pounds. Get the difference? This way, you're encouraged to keep going and stick with those healthy habits. If you reward yourself for the reward instead (in this case for losing 10 pounds), you might find yourself choosing some very unhealthy routes to losing weight. You don't want to encourage unhealthy behavior, do you? So reward yourself for good behavior and not for the results of the good behavior.

Whatever reward you settle on let it be something that matters to you. It doesn't matter if someone else thinks your reward is silly. For example, when I finish writing a chapter, I light a vanilla and cinnamon scented candle. I do it because it feels like I'm in heaven. It's amazing. It feels good to me. Is it silly? Oh probably. But it works.

Once you've done the thing you set out to do, make sure you reward yourself instantly or as soon as you can. Say you love flavored sparkling water. Did you just finish a workout? You can immediately reward yourself with that! Of course, I assume the water has 0 calories, so you don't invalidate your workout or DASH diet plan. If you delay the reward, then you will have a harder time of using the reward to encourage your good behavior.

Now you might be as smart as Einstein but I'm going to pull out ahead of you and issue this warning: don't you ever reward yourself before you have accomplished your goal. I mean I guess it seems like there would be some sort of logic to reverse-engineering the behavior-reward process, but it won't work. You'll just undermine yourself. I also have to add if you know in your heart that you didn't earn a reward then don't give yourself one. Be honest with yourself. No one's giving you points for getting rewards. You owe yourself some honesty.

It's A Bad Day, not A Bad Life

There will be times when life happens, and for some reason or the other you don't achieve what you set out to do. Let me say this right now: just because you didn't achieve your goal doesn't mean you're an utter failure.

Setbacks happen. It's normal to relapse. You can't control everything. You can control your response, though. Just because you skipped a day of workouts does not mean it's back to square one. Just because you caved and got that Snickers bar does not mean you've undone all your hard work. You can always get back in the saddle. Look at all you've achieved so far and let that spur you on.

Learn not to beat yourself up for the setbacks. It's a waste of energy and quite frankly a tad silly.

You're not going to gain 20 pounds because you ate that chocolate you shouldn't have. Get back to the plan and to crushing your goals! You're not a failure. You're human, and you had a human moment. Now you can either wallow in self-loathing or pick yourself up and get back to dancing like you never tripped and fell to begin with.

Practical Goal-Setting

Now you know you need to set SMART goals which you can chunk down even further. You know how to incorporate rewards into your goals. Now I want you to practice this. That old cliché is true - practice makes perfect.

To make the DASH diet work for you, we're going to set some goals to help you better manage your weight.

Step one. What's a behavior you regularly engage in that you really want to change? Think about it.

Step two. Set a goal which deals with this behavior. Keep your focus on the behavior and a goal you can achieve within the short-term.

Step three. Write the goal down, starting with the words "I will" to get the most effect.

Step four. Remember to keep the goal SMART. Once again that's Specific, Measurable, Action-oriented, Realistic, and Timed.

You can apply this process towards your DASH diet, your workouts and other areas in life.

Chapter Eight Conscious Eating

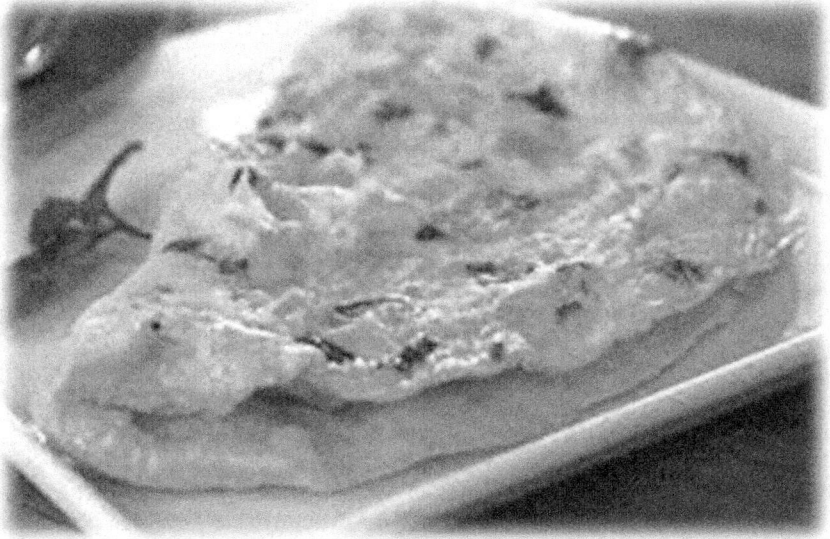

Let's talk about conscious eating. What even is that? No one can eat unless they're conscious, right? Wrong. A lot of people eat without thinking about what they're eating and why they're eating. They just get a sudden craving for something make a call and place the order. It arrives they plop themselves down on the couch and proceed to shovel the food down their pie holes while watching 13 Reasons Why.

When I talk about conscious eating, I mean being completely immersed in the moment as you eat. You know what it is you're putting in your body. You know why you're choosing to eat this and not that. You know when it's time to put the fork down. When you eat consciously, you will find it easier to lose weight since you're more in tune with your body and the emotions which may or may not be behind the desire for you to eat.

Our bodies are constantly talking to us all the time letting us know what it is we need. However, we've gotten used to merely eating for taste and not nutrition. Rather than eat to live, we live to eat. You don't believe me? All you have to do is walk into your favorite fast food restaurant and see the ungodly proportions being served. Why would you need that much? It's eating for the sake of it and not because

160

you need all that food.

So let's get honest right now. Are you the kind of person who eats without thinking? Do you eat as you drive or walk? Do you eat while you watch TV or read? Do you eat while doing something other than you know eating? If you answered yes, then we've got some work to do buddy. That needs to stop. Think carefully about the last time you did nothing but focus on you and your food as you ate. When was the last time you really tasted the food? Don't feel bad about it. We're just going to change that. We're going to pick up a new good habit. The habit of conscious eating.

How Conscious Eating Helps

When you eat consciously you tend to slow down the speed you eat at. When you eat slowly, you give your body time to let you know when you're full. Chances are you'll be full before you even finish what's on your plate. When you rush your food, you don't realize when you eat past your capacity. Ever felt incredibly bloated after a meal? Chances are you ate too much too fast.

Anyone who eats too fast will struggle with losing the pounds. That's just the way it happens.

When you eat fast, you don't give your brain enough time to let you know "Hey buddy we're good here. Put the fork down now." It usually takes about 20 minutes after you start eating for your brain to realize you're full. So when you eat too fast, you get too stuffed, and it just feels plain horrible. The fix? Eat slowly and mindfully.

Conscious eating also allows you to have better relationships with your loved ones and friends.

How so? See when you're always munching mindlessly while watching something on TV, it's easy to not engage with the people around you. However, when you and your loved ones make a habit of turning off all distractions during mealtimes you'll find your relationships and friendships are that much strengthened. You'll find you all share a much deeper connection than you've ever experienced before. This reason alone makes conscious eating worth it in my book.

When you eat mindfully, you're more aware of the

flavors. Your food tastes way better than if you simply scarf it down! How's that for another benefit? As you savor your food you get to really enjoy it. Also savoring means eating small amounts slowly. As a result, you might find yourself full before you're even halfway done.

Imagine you're following the DASH diet and eating mindfully as well. You'll get to enjoy your food without punishing yourself for eating. Best of all you'll lose even more weight and develop a better connection between your body and your mind.

How to Feel More Sated

It's not hard to achieve the feeling of satiety when you follow a few simple guidelines.

Remember how I said it takes your brain at least 20 minutes to realize you're full? How can you take advantage of this so that you eat less?

Eat slow. It's not a race. This isn't Man versus Food. Take your time to chew.

Drink something nice and warm before you eat. You'll feel a lot fuller faster. You could just have a glass of water before every meal. I guarantee you'll find it hard to go overboard with the food.

Eat your veggies. Lots of them. They'll fill you up really good and don't have as much calories as their volume. Try to add in the kind of veggies that force you to really chew.

Put down the fork every now and then as you eat.

Why Do You Eat?

I once went on a 7-day water fast. I had nothing but water and some electrolytes. Not the mix which would have something to sweeten it. Just pure water, Himalayan pink salt, and potassium chloride. Don't ask. That's not the subject of this book.

Here's what I found particularly interesting: I had never truly been hungry until I did that fast. Not once in my life. Am I saying I'll never used the words "I'm hungry" prior to those 7 days? No. I'm saying I realized I had never experienced true hunger.

Think about it. When you eat, is it because it's lunch?

Or because it's dinner? Or because you've got some food in the fridge? When you eat is it because there's still something on your plate and you believe it shouldn't go to waste, so you just keep eating? Sometimes - in fact, I'd say a lot of the time - everyone eats just because "it's time."

Other times we eat because our emotions tell us to. Feeling anxious? Eat something. Feeling exhilarated about just getting paid? Eat something. Feeling angry and upset? Eat something.

Just got a promotion? Eat something to celebrate. See a lot of the time negative and positive emotions trigger us into eating even though we're not hungry!

So how do you keep yourself from eating when you're not feeling hunger? You can start by getting in touch with how your body feels. Get in touch with your gut. The next time you want to reach for a snack or a meal you know you shouldn't have just ask yourself: "Do I feel hungry physically?" Take a moment to really check in with your second brain (which is your gut). "Am I hungry, or would it simply be nice to pop insert-random-food-here into my mouth?"

Once you begin to consciously keep track of yourself like this, you'll find yourself giving in less and less to eating for the sake of eating. Just make a commitment to yourself right here right now that you're not going to eat unless you're hungry. This is where mindful conscious eating will help you. Since you gain a better appreciation for food while eating mindfully you're less likely to open your fridge and fix yourself something when you don't need it.

Dealing With Cravings

How do you deal with cravings for unhealthy fattening food? One key thing that would help is making sure you don't have easy access to those foods. In other words, I want you to inventory your fridge, freezer, and pantry. Anything that does not line up with the DASH diet has simply got to go. No room for negotiations, my friend. Not if you want to achieve success and maintain your goals as well.

I wish dealing with cravings was as easy as simply cleaning out your food stores, but there's so much more to it. There will be times where you'll be faced

166

with the challenge of indulging in your favorite guilty treat and you'll go out of your way to make it happen. How do you best handle those really challenging times? Here are a few practical tips to help you out.

Liquids.

Rather than eat your weight in something that will make you feel sick and guilty try finding a drink that works best for you. You could try some decaffeinated tea. There's a whole slew of flavors out there from very good brands. Not a fan of tea? Fine. Try some low-cal hot cocoa instead. Not in the mood? I personally love ice cold fizzy water. It gives me a nice full feeling and the tingle in my mouth when I drink it is just heavenly. Whatever you do, alcohol is a no-no. Don't use it to satisfy your cravings. It packs a lot of calories and quite frankly can mess up your commitment to eating and living better. Also, it's not worth all the sleep problems it causes.

Black screens Specifically your TV screens. I wish I could show you how badly TV can numb your mind and make you a lot more susceptible to eating a lot of crap. You're in even greater danger of being triggered to eat when the fast food commercials come on. How do you stop TV from triggering you into poor eating choices? Just turn it off. Watch it a lot less. Got a program you absolutely have to watch? Then you could just mute the TV each time another food commercial comes on. Find other activities you can enjoy that don't revolve around the tube.

Brush your teeth.

You already know you should do this at least twice a day. I'll go so far as to ask you to brush after each meal - provided you're not suffering from teeth sensitivity issues.

Don't just brush. Get some mint floss and get in between those pearly whites of yours. It's been proven that the last thing you want to do after cleaning your teeth is to eat. So keep your mouth clean.

Get busy.

Sean Paul really was on to something with that song. When you're busy doing something with your hands, you can't put things in your mouth. Unless you're an alien. So find a way to keep your hands and your mind busy. Busy yourself with things and projects that are interesting to you. I can't count how many times I get so immersed in a project that I don't remember I haven't had anything to eat in hours!

Snack healthy.

Let's face it: snacks are awesome. Am I right? They're not quite a meal yet they're just wonderful to have. If you're going to have a snack you might as well prepare healthy ones. Think of all the junk food that you love and try to think up healthy alternatives.

Can't figure anything out? Who's your pal? Google. Also, when you find alternatives which work great plan ahead. This way, when the craving hits you, you're ready to take it on.

Eat enough.

Follow the meal plan and you're less likely to be up at night scavenging for food.

If you've had just the right amount of food for the day, you won't get hit with random cravings at night when you should be preparing for bed.

Nap.

Can you eat while you sleep? You can? My goodness... I guess this tip is not for you. I also badly want to know how you do that without choking to death. For those who can't eat while sleeping - meaning the rest of us normies - napping is a great way to get over the craving.

Cravings like hunger tend to come in waves. A great way to wait it out if you're not too busy is to take a nice nap.

Gum.

Go sugar-free. It's a great way to keep your mouth moving without packing on calories.

Also, it doesn't hurt that there are so many wonderful flavors out there to try. Gum is your best friend for keeping cravings at bay.

Get mindful.

You know how to do that now. You know how to check in with your body and see what it really needs if anything. So each time you feel a craving coming on ask yourself if you really want or need that. Check in with yourself, and you'll feel the craving pass more often than not.

Chapter Nine Eating Your Emotions

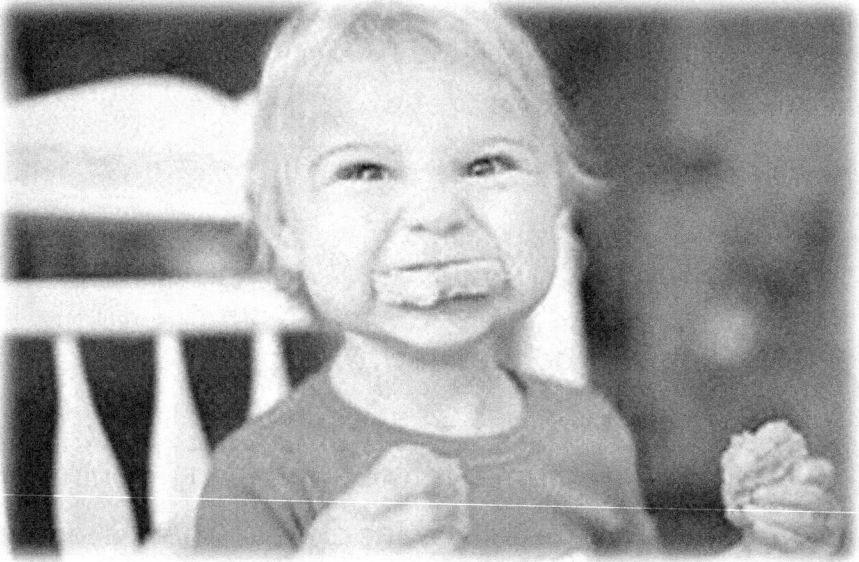

We've talked a bit about emotion-triggered eating, but we're going to really sink our teeth into this topic now. Are you the sort of person who grabs the phone to order a pizza or a burger or something even though you're not actually hungry? Do you tend to get yourself some food depending on your emotions? Did you answer "yes" to these questions? Well then you are an emotional eater. No sugar-coating it.

Emotional eaters will usually scarf down large amounts of food at once. No, it's hardly ever the healthy stuff. It's food laden with calories and fat and all other kinds of things that don't do your body any good. Basically, emotional eaters reach for "comfort" food when they start to get "the feels." It's a way of dealing with emotions that you don't want to face for whatever reason. This is one dragon you're going to have to slay if you want long term success following the DASH way of eating.

Why Do We Do It?

Emotional eating happens when there are emotions you just can't and won't face. A lot of the time, you remain blissfully unaware of the way your emotions are connected to your eating choices and habits.

173

There's so much to be said against emotional eating. It's not just the fact that you'll have to deal with more and more pounds on your gut thighs and everywhere else. It's that when you stuff your face full of unhealthy gunk, and you make a habit of it, it's easy to eat less of the healthy stuff. Eating less of the healthy stuff means your body isn't getting the nutrition it needs to properly function. You're at risk for injuries and all sorts of diseases. When you get hit with a disease, your body is not fully equipped to beat it because it has the wrong fuel.

Why do we eat our emotions rather than deal with them? It's not hard to see how we can fall into this trap. See growing up, we learn that a little food can make us feel loads better. What's the first thing that happens as a baby when you begin wailing? Mummy tries to give you some food if she hasn't already. What happens when you get good grades? Daddy will take you to your favorite ice cream place. What happens when something doesn't turn out the way you'd have liked? Your uncle tries to distract you or make you feel better by offering you some sweet treat.

As time flies by and we get older, we hold on to these

habits. We use the food as a coping mechanism whenever we're feeling stressed out. We use the food to celebrate whenever something great just happened. Do you see now how easy it is to be an emotional eater? Don't beat yourself up. Today's society is just set up in such a way as to encourage emotional eating.

What Sets You Off?

If you're going to beat this thing, you need to know what drives you to eat in the first place. There are all sorts of triggers for emotional eating. Boredom, anger, depression, stress, anxiety, relationship issues, work issues, depression frustration, and low self-worth are just a few of the many things which can set off the habit. If you find that you're usually set off by these feelings, don't worry. We're going to deal with this. You'll learn that the fridge does not hold all the answers to your problems.

What are your own triggers? If you're going to get a lid on this bad habit, then you need to know what sets you off. Get into the habit of keeping a food log. Log

175

your meals and log the way you felt as you ate. You want to do this especially when you eat too much.

You also should consult a professional therapist or counselor so they can help you to identify your triggers better and to break the hold emotional eating has on your life. Before you head off to find a good licensed counselor, I'm going to give you a few tips that have helped me along my journey too. Yes, I've been there before. So I get it! We're in this together. Here's some stuff you can try which all fall under one umbrella.

Get Distracted.

Tempted to reach for that snack you don't need? Try anything else. Go take a nice long luxurious bath. Go for a swim. Take a walk. Phone a friend and talk about how much you're craving whatever you're craving. Just talking about it takes the pressure off and the craving passes easily after that. You could read a good book, play a video game, or go for a walk in the park. Drink a glass or two of water and chew some sugar-free gum for good measure. Go mow the lawn. Listen to your favorite music or an audiobook. Deliberately relax. This is a great alternative to dealing with the stress, which triggers your emotional eating. You get the idea. If there's anything that can help distract you from your cravings caused by the feelings, do it.

Meditate.

Meditation is amazing. With constant practice, you'll find yourself very much in touch with your feelings. You'll be able to face them without fear. You'll see your cravings for what they are and just allow them flutter by like butterflies. That's the power of meditation.

How to Know for Sure if You're an Emotional Eater Look, I'm willing to bet there isn't a person on the planet who hasn't had something to eat or drink simply out of sheer boredom. Emotional eating is something nearly everyone has dealt with.

It's just that for some people it's more serious than just reaching for a Twinkie when they're bored. How do you know you've got a major problem on your hands?

If you're an emotional eater:

You eat super fast. The feel and flavor of the food don't register when you eat.

You eat ridiculously huge amounts of food when you're nowhere near hungry.

You tend to hide your food and your eating habits because you know those are things you'll be embarrassed about if others could see you.

You eat until you feel like you're about to burst.

Does any of that hit a little too close to home? Then please seek professional counsel. You've got this. I believe in you.

Chapter Ten Seek Help

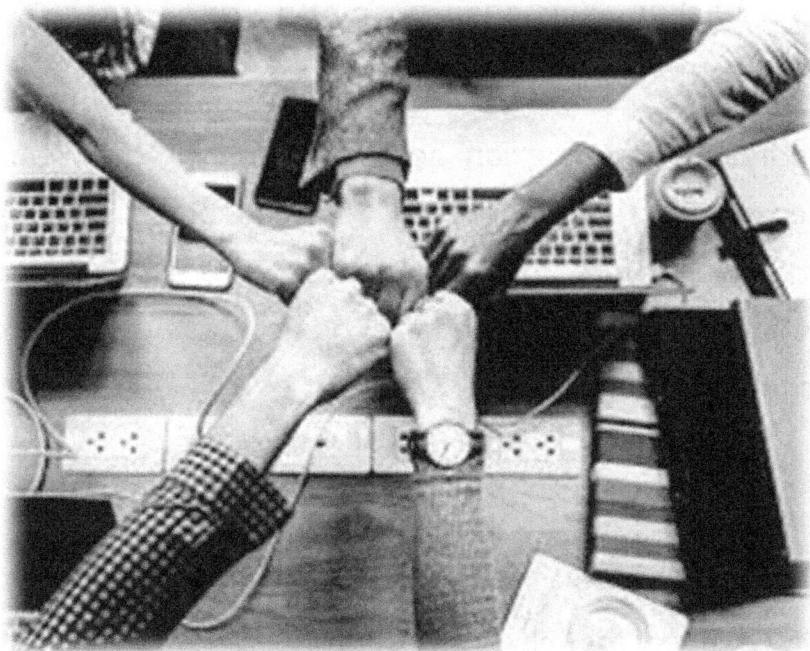

If there's one thing that I've come to believe it's that weight-loss is a journey that's easier to go when you're not alone. If you want to make the changes you need to get the results you want then you'll need some backup. You need people in your corner. You need help along the way.

Family and friends can be there for you. You could even get some support from your colleagues at work. No matter where you have to draw that support from get it, and you're going to achieve your weight-loss targets.

At Home

Before all others, chances are your friends and family are the ones who are going to be the most supportive of your ambitions. How do you get them to help you out? Make it clear to them your intention to follow the DASH diet plan. Call up a meeting of your loved ones! Make it clear to them that if they won't support you actively, they at least need to respect your plans. You'll be surprised to find that there may be a few of your friends and family who have been thinking about making the same changes!

Let them know how much you'll appreciate them cheering you on as you move to this new way of eating. With great friends and family, you'll find the support you receive to be overwhelming. In a good way, of course.

Let your friends and family know the best ways to help you achieve your weight loss goals as you embark on this DASH diet journey. Let them know you'd rather that they encourage you for good behavior rather than constant criticism when you slip up every now and then.

You can (and should) have a food and workout log. Better than that, you can put this log on the fridge, or somewhere everyone can see it. Why would you want to put yourself out there like that you ask? It's simply, so everyone remembers what your targets are. It's also a great way to keep them proactive about helping you lose the pounds successfully.

Another great thing to try is to set some money aside for every time you make healthy decisions which lead toward your goal. Once you hit one of your goals (say losing 20 pounds in 6 weeks), you could take the money and splurge on a nice reward for yourself and your family and friends who have been in your corner all through! Just make sure the reward is not centered around food so you can stay on track.

Has your family decided they have nothing to change about their diet and activity levels? No problem. What you can do is clear a section of the fridge pantry and freezer where you can keep your DASH approved food items. Be very clear that everyone keeps the junk food in a different section entirely. Try to be nice about it, please.

At Work

Family is great, and friends are awesome. However, chances are you spend a lot of your time at work, so it only makes sense to let your colleagues in on the changes you're making too. This way it's easier to not have them unwittingly sabotage you. You'd also be pleasantly surprised to find that there are a number of your colleagues who are equally interested in losing some weight as well You may meet each of your colleagues and let them know of your goals nice as you please.

Don't be a jerk about it. Let them know you'd love it if they could help you out and encourage you any way they can. If you have especially understanding coworkers, you can try to get them to bring less or no junk food into the office. Do you constantly have work during lunches? Try to get them to throw in some restaurants with healthy options and great salad bars.

What to Do When People Are Challenging

You're not going to get along with everyone. That's just a fact of life. If you run into someone or people who go out of their way to tempt you into having some food that's not part of your plan, then what do you do?

Let me point out that not everyone is deliberately out to get you. Some people genuinely don't realize how their actions are subverting your weight loss goals. They might bring you some food just as a gift or a simple, thoughtful gesture. They might bring in the wrong foods which cause your mouth to water and your resolve to quiver.

Whether you're dealing with someone who's deliberately trying to sabotage your efforts or someone who's doing this unwittingly here are a few things you could try.

Have a rehearsed response ready for those who offer you food.

I mean write out an actual script which will be the response you give them. Get in front of a mirror and rehearse it. When dealing with these sorts of people, you only need to learn to keep saying no each time they entreat you with some delicious donuts or cookies or something. The more ready you are to handle a tempting situation like that the more likely you'll be able to stand your ground.

What kind of responses could you give the next time you're plied with food? You could say, "It looks delicious, but I'm so stuffed I can't eat anymore." Or a simple "No thanks, I'm good." Make your script

184

yours and use it when you find yourself cornered by that one person who just wants you to have "just one bite."

If you have to visit this person or these people at their home you can let them know before you get there that you will not be eating. If you can help it though it might be best to avoid seeing them altogether especially if they've repeatedly ignored your requests that they help you make healthier eating choices.

Are they simply not giving you any way out? Are things starting to look very awkward? You could just take the food they're offering. What's the catch? Don't eat it. Throw it out or better yet give it to someone who looks like they could use a free meal.

Chapter Eleven Your Questions Answered

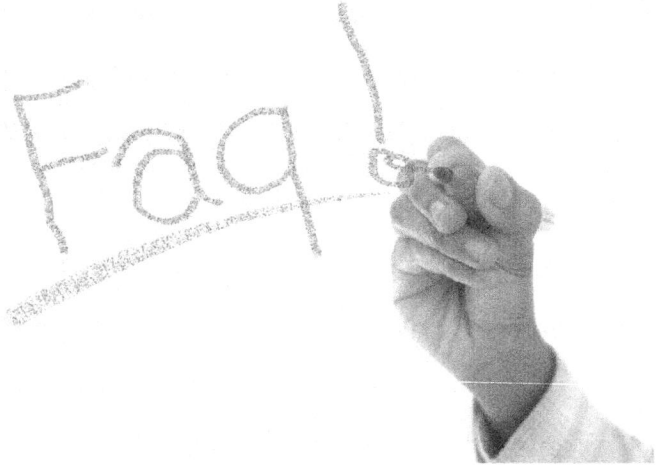

So you've made it this far into the book. Perhaps you've already started on the DASH way of living. If so I congratulate you.

You might however still be hesitant to get your feet wet. I understand that. You have concerns.

Questions which need answering. To allay your fears once and for all, I'm going to cover some of what you want to know. I'm willing to repeat myself because I badly don't want you to give up.

You can lose weight. You can keep it off. You just have to keep an open mind.

Why should I buy into the DASH diet when tonnes of diets have proven themselves useless?

I understand that you'd still be pretty skeptical about this. There is just way too much information out there that it's become hard to pick out what's the real deal and what isn't. You have people who are non-experts in health talking about this or that diet - which they haven't had any first hand experience with. I've already mentioned that the DASH diet has gone through clinical trials with large samples of people and all with tremendous results. If you find that hard to believe, then believe me. Why did I even start writing this book? I realized there was a very serious need out there. People are seeking answers for better ways to achieve the best versions of themselves. Yet with the barrage of information coming at them, it's hard to see which path to take. I wrote this because I did it myself, and I got results. I would never endorse something I have not personally tested. That's just how I roll. In the end, for you to really be sure, I recommend you check in with your doctor and nutritionist so they can give you the best advice on whether or not the DASH diet is worth trying.

I'm not big on fruits and definitely don't care for veggies. How am I supposed to follow the DASH diet?

Would you be more willing to open your mind to fruits and veggies if I told you that people who don't eat enough of those foods are the ones who battle the most with their weight? If you really want results at least give this a go. You have nothing to lose and just might find that you'll come to love fruits and veggies. There are ways to spruce up your meals, and I've already given you a fantastic meal plan to work with. Eating healthy doesn't have to be a bore or a chore. A diet that's rich in veggies will definitely help you lose the weight.

I know veggies and fruits are good for me, but I barely think about stocking up on them.

How do I fix this?

Make a list before you go grocery shopping. Make it a fun plan to try out every vegetable there is available. This way, you can find out which ones are your favorite. Give it enough time, and you'll be craving them!

To get more veggies in your diet, you can also consider incorporating them into meals like your morning omelet. Need a way to get the fruit in? Add them to your cereal. Make a habit of packing fruits and veggies with you when you head out to work or wherever.

Dining out? Hit the salad bar. There are so many delicious amazing salads you can try especially when you're in a good restaurant. If you don't feel like making your own salads, this is a great alternative!

Always put your fruits and veggies within sight. You want them to be just an arm's length away.

You can place them on your kitchen counter. Got some in the fridge? Set it up, so they're right in front of you when you open it. Why? When you can see your fruits and veggies, you're more likely to eat them.

Be sure to stock up on all sorts of fresh, frozen, and canned fruits and vegetables so you can enjoy them weekly. Remember your veggies make up most of your meals, so the last thing you want to do is run out.

How do I tell which fruit and veggies are good and fresh? And how do I store them?

Easy. Look for veggies and fruit which aren't shriveled don't look bruised don't have mold and don't seem slimy. Also, smell is a good way to tell if something

190

isn't fresh. Does it smell off like it's going bad? Then don't buy it. You could also enlist the help of the store workers to help you decide which items to go for. You could request info on storing the fruits and veggies you go for.

When it comes to most veggies, you can't really buy a stockpile of them. Same with fruits. If you're not using all of it within the next few days or at least within the week, they're likely to go bad. So make sure you only buy enough to last you some days. If you want fruits and veggies which will keep longer then stock up on the frozen kind.

When you're shopping, make sure you keep the fruit and veggies on top of everything else in your cart. If you put heavy stuff on it some of the fruit will bruise and the vegetables will suffer for it too.

At home keep as much of your produce in the crisper compartment of your fridge so they can keep longer. Got some already cut veggies and fruits? Keep them in the fridge.

Rather than wash your veggies and fruit before putting them away, opt to wash them right before you eat or use them instead. This is so they stay as fresh as they can for as long as possible.

If you've got some unripe fruits you need to put them in a brown paper bag (make sure it's only closed loosely). Better yet get a ripening bowl. Why does this matter? The gases they give off as they ripen, encourage more ripening. If you'll like them to ripen faster, you can put a ripe apple or banana in the brown bag or the ripening bowl along with the rest of the fruit.

Everyone says carbs make you add weight. Why are they part of the DASH diet?

Not all carbs are created equal. I don't consider carbs all that bad in moderation. However, if you're trying to lose weight, then you should be concerned about the fact that you're eating carbs. When you think of carbs, you probably think of bread white rice and pasta. Guess what?

Fruits are carbs. Veggies are carbs too.

So what makes the difference? If you're trying to lose

weight and eat right then you'll find carbs which have fiber and lots of other great nutrients are good for you. I'm talking about whole grains, veggies, and fruit. They're packed with phytochemicals, minerals and lots of vitamins. Also, these carbs are the complex kind. Yes, they still break down into sugar like the simple carbs, but because of their complexity, they do so slowly. As a result, our blood sugar levels do not spike hard and fast like when you eat plain sugar. So it's safe to have these carbs – lentils, beans, whole grains, and veggies.

It's hard to do the DASH diet when I'm on the road. Any advice?

Yes, it's going to be a bit more challenging when you're on the move to focus on your DASH meal plan. You're going to have to try. First things first control your portions, so you're not eating too much. Find an option that works with the DASH diet. If you can't find options, then really control your portions as best as you can.

Also, it's more important than ever that you stick with

your exercise routine. You need to be active as often as you can. Take time to explore where you are on foot. Take the stairs when you can. Go hiking. Hit the gym if you're lodged in a hotel. Do whatever you can to move your body!

Conclusion

We've come to the end, my friends. I've given you the tools you need to get in the best shape of your life. The choice is yours whether you choose to follow through and succeed or choose to remain in your comfort zone.

Remember all you need to focus on is just today. Just start. Make this your new life and you'll be glad you did.

Here's to the new you!